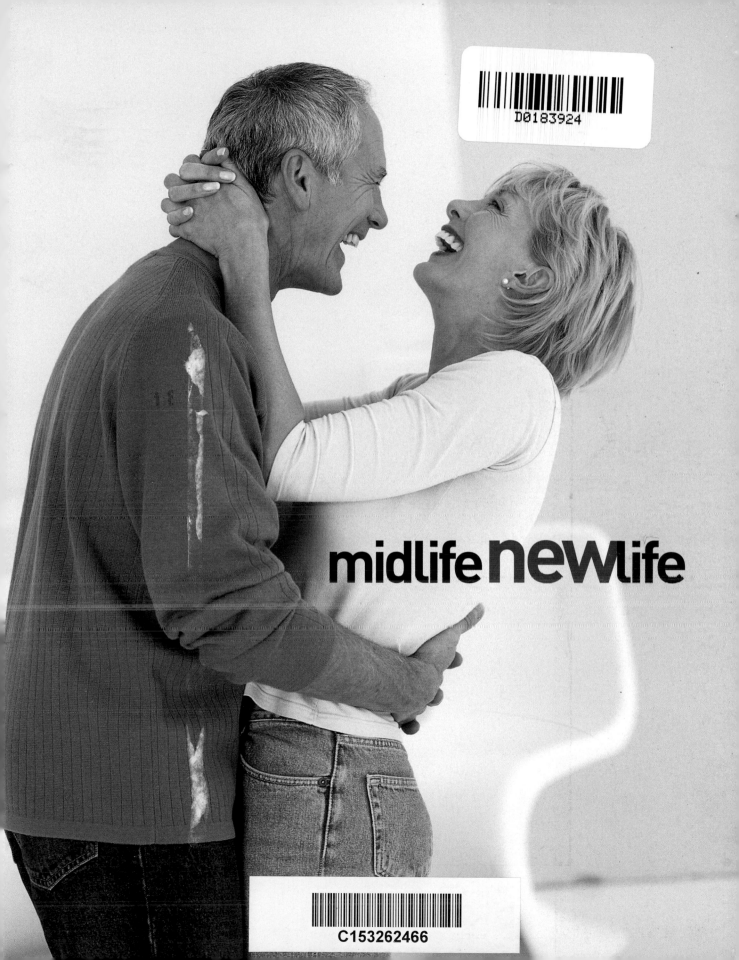

midlife **new**life

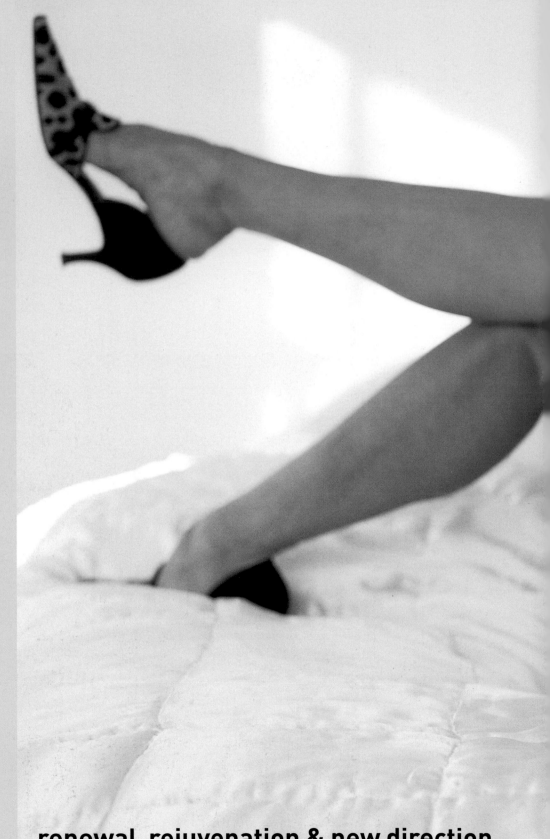

Quadrille   **renewal, rejuvenation & new direction**

Judith Wills

special photography by **Liz McAulay**

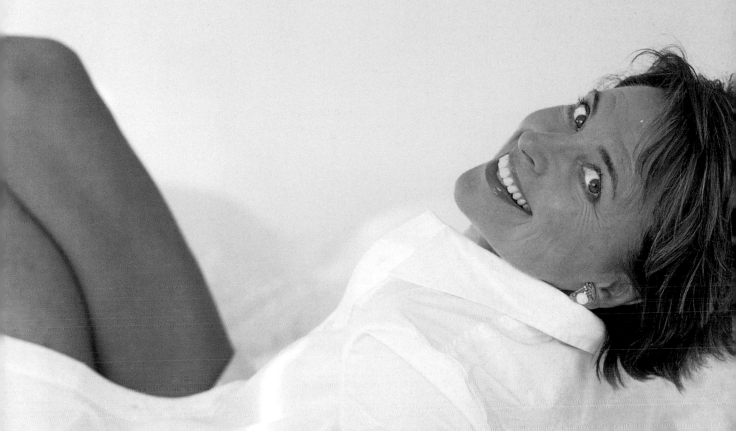

midlife
newlife

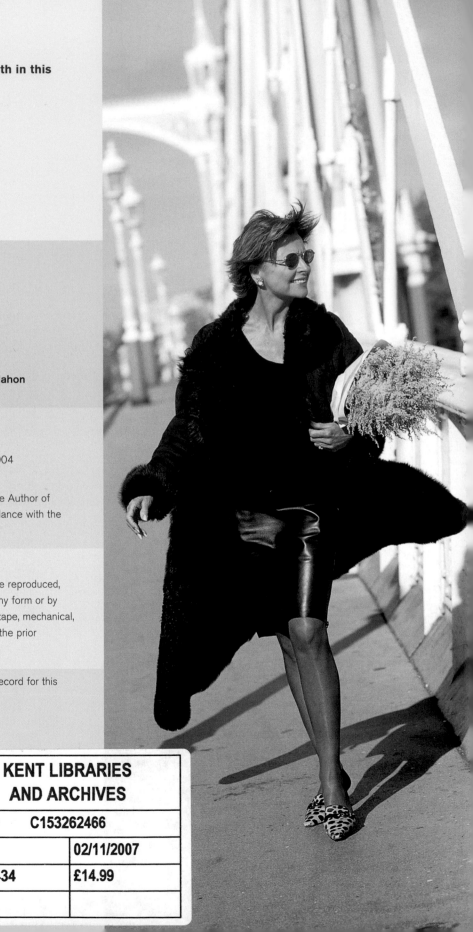

To Tony, the inspiration for much, both in this book and in my life

First published in 2004 by
Quadrille Publishing Limited,
Alhambra House,
27–31 Charing Cross Road,
London WC2H OLS

This paperback edition first published in 2005
Reprinted in 2005
10 9 8 7 6 5 4 3 2

Editorial Director **Jane O'Shea**
Editor & Project Manager **Lewis Esson**
Art Director **Mary Evans**
Production **Jane Rogers**
Illustration **Bridget Bodoano**
Photography **Liz McAulay**
Styling **Claire Roberts**
Make-up **Dottie Monaghan** and **James McMahon**

1 84400 092 3 Hardback
1 84400 144 X Paperback

Printed in China

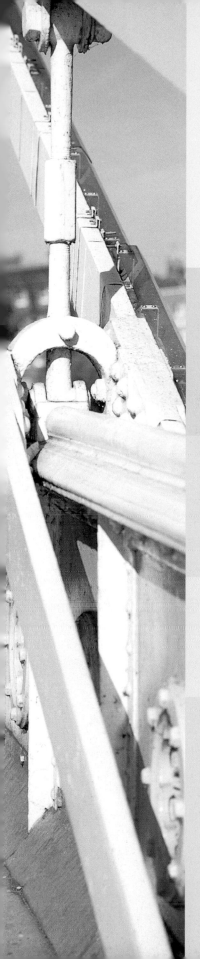

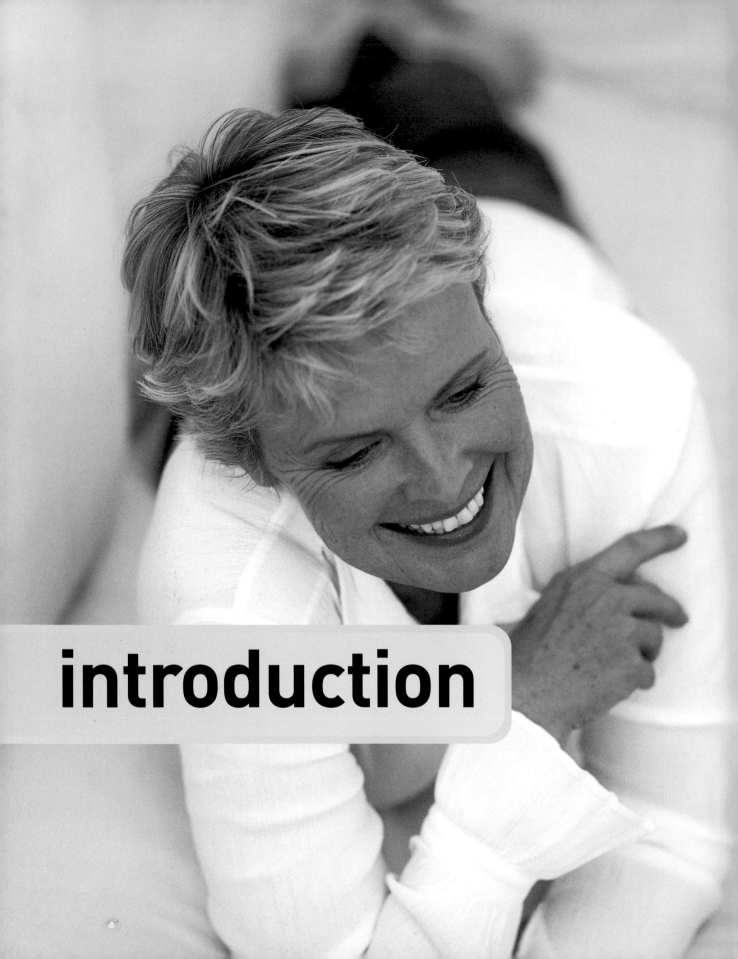

introduction

Mid life...You... Can you believe it? Well – DID you ever really think you'd reach half a century or so? I certainly didn't – but I got there, somehow!

This book aims to prove that being 'middle-aged' is no reason for depression and may even be a cause for celebration – the start of your new life. I have tried hard not to offer false hope of a return to the physical fitness or shape of youth, or to peddle miracle cures to keep you alive, fertile or wrinkle-free to 150. However, I firmly believe – and know – that everything you don't like about yourself can be improved, all the baggage that comes with no longer being 20 can be a blessing not a deadweight, and that at any time from your late forties through to your sixties you can, if you choose, begin the most fulfilling – even exciting – decades of your life.

As we are all living longer than ever before, you've got at least forty or fifty years of good (in its best sense) living ahead, with a bit of luck. And we 'baby-boomers' are lucky in that many of us do have better health, healthier finances and more opportunities than any other generation before us.

In *Mid Life, New Life*, I have set out to make the most of this good fortune. I wanted to document all that can realistically be achieved once we are no longer in the state known as youth; to encourage you to try what is documented and, most importantly, to tell the truth. From food to physical fitness, from health to libido and emotions, if you need guidance and motivation I hope you will find them here.

Judith Wills

January 2004

fuel for your newlife

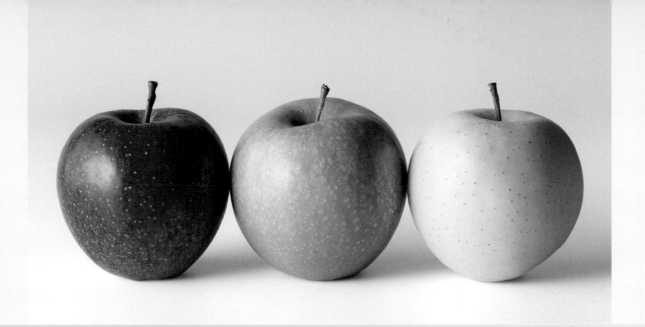

Food is fundamental to our total well-being, health and existence. What we eat IS at least some of what we are – which is why I describe food as 'fuel'.

Although there are other influences on how good you feel, how long you live and how healthy you are, the right fuel is certainly one of the most important factors in defining how well you function.

In Section 1, we will be looking at all the ways in which the right body fuel is empowering. In mid life, a good diet is especially relevant. It may be time to alter long-standing food habits that aren't serving you well. Time to prime your body for the inevitable changes of the years ahead.

Certainly, the ideas that we discuss here should enhance your life, not hamper it. Good food and drink are not only priorities – but pleasures. Don't miss out.

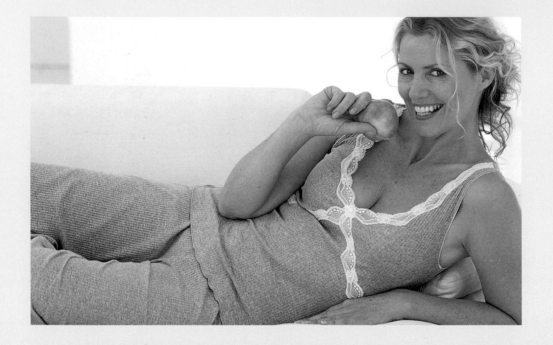

what do you eat? Your diet makes a difference to your life in so many ways.

How do you feel today? How do you feel this very minute? How will you feel next week, next year – or in ten or twenty years' time? Believe it or not, immediate, short-term and long-term health and well-being are, to a surprising degree, governed by what you eat and drink (and, of course, by what you don't).

A good diet – together with adequate exercise – is among the most important markers of a healthy and long life. Yet only in recent years has this been recognized by 'officialdom', from the World Health Organization through national government health departments, and finally the message is being accepted by every one of us. We are what we eat.

Knowing the message and finding the motivation to act on it are different matters. In this section, Fuel for Your New Life, we offer that motivation by looking in detail at how a good diet can effect sometimes almost miraculous improvements in so many areas of our well-being.

We look at how the physical and mental ageing process is affected by food, and at how the major diseases of the twenty-first century – such as cancers, heart disease, diabetes, high blood pressure and arthritis – can be kept at bay. Of course, we are all different, and you will find out how to get an optimum diet whether you are 40, 50 or 60. Find out the truth about antioxidants and check out how many of the Top 20 Anti-ageing Foods appear regularly in your diet. Eat with an eye on your looks, because skin, hair, eyes and 'sparkle' can all improve.

Few people feel their best when they are carrying a few kilos that weren't there a decade ago. Find out the truth about middle-age spread and dieting at 40-plus, and get practical help on dealing with cellulite and hard-to-shift fat, lumps and bumps.

Does detoxing really work? IS there actually such a thing? We look at the facts behind all the detox myths and help you decide whether a detox plan could work for you. Our effective but gentle programme gives you the benefits of detoxing without any unwanted side-effects.

Around the age of 50, diet becomes a major factor for many women in beating the negative symptoms of the menopause, and we provide everything you need to know – from eating to help minimize hot flushes and headaches to increasing energy and libido.

There really are 'brain foods' that can help you retain your powers of concentration, memory and sharpness. We look at helping you to optimum brain power through not only eating the right foods and avoiding the wrong ones, but by eating the right foods at the right times.

This section offers a variety of eating plans from which you can select to suit your own needs. Whichever plan you do choose, enjoyment of your menus should be a top priority. So here is a special plea – take time to find real pleasure in your menu planning and food shopping, even if you are only preparing meals for yourself. Buy the best-quality foods you can, enjoy cooking and savour every mouthful. For busy mid-lifers who have spent many years too busy to cook or too busy making meals for others to really enjoy food - now is the time to start.

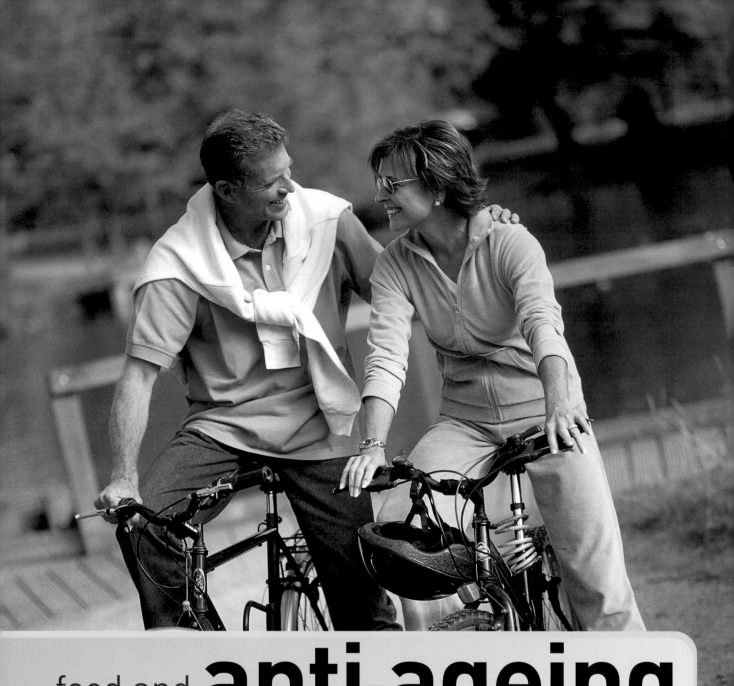

food and anti-ageing

The quality and length of your life, and your appearance and health as you age, can, to a large extent, be governed by you – and the decisions you make about what to eat and drink will form a very important part of the picture. Happily, it is never too late to start making those decisions the right ones.

Research shows that up to 75% of the ageing process is not genetic. In other words, how well you age is largely under your own control. Diet is an important component of this self-help anti-ageing process. The typical signs of ageing – the onset of conditions like cancer, heart disease or diabetes, decline in general health and vitality, the appearance of wrinkles and changes in hair and skin texture – can be kept at bay by a good diet or exacerbated by a poor one.

What you eat can not only slow down the speed at which you age, but to a certain extent can also turn back the clock – actually helping you to look and feel younger. Although this is not usually a fast process, you should notice certain improvements, such as increased energy or better skin, within as little as a week. Improvements in health – for example, a reduction in joint pain, tiredness or blood pressure – may take from weeks to months.

First we look at eating right from early mid life, around forty, through the fifties and into your sixties. Knowing what to eat and what not to eat – and choosing the right foods for energy – is important whatever your age, but the optimum mix of foods can vary according to your current decade.

Most people have heard the words 'antioxidants' and 'phytochemicals', but many are unsure of how these help, or even what they are. We help you make sense of these potent plant components and list the Top 20 Anti-ageing Foods.

Later in the chapter you will find specific advice for keeping your looks – skin, eyes, hair and so on – in good condition, and finally there is a choice of diet plans, one of which will be your own blueprint for anti-ageing.

eat for your age

around 40

The early 40s are a hectic few years for most people – with children still at home, a career still in need of complete focus, personal relationships to maintain. Juggling time is an every-day necessity – and when life is that busy, healthy eating may be the last thing on your mind.

However, a few simple dietary tips can help you feel much better, give you more energy, help you sleep better and beat the small, but often long-term, symptoms of ill health that can result from stress, or simply the beginnings of getting older.

how to eat
A speedy but nourishing breakfast is vital every day, to help your brain and body work better. Research shows that people who skip breakfast perform more poorly in the morning, that they lack concentration and they may feel dizzy due to low blood sugar.

Breakfast should include some complex carbs (e.g. whole-meal bread, whole-grain cereal), some protein (e.g. egg, yoghurt, milk) a little fat (present in many protein foods and also in butter or spread), and nuts and seeds – excellent foods in their own right (see the Top 20 Anti-ageing Foods, pages 20–23). The Diet Plan for Your 40s (see page 28) includes suggestions for quick and easy breakfasts of this type.

Lunch should be reasonably low in carbohydrate and high in protein, as research shows that this will produce the best afternoon performance – too much carb will slow you down and can make you feel drowsy. Thus a chicken salad or fish and vegetables is better than two rounds of sandwiches or a plate of pasta. Again, you will find quick lunch ideas in the diet plans.

Around 5–6pm you should get a small snack to restore your energy – an apple and a small piece of cheese, a yoghurt, or some fresh nuts are ideal energy foods which will keep your blood sugar level constant while you travel home from work, deal with children's meals or have to work late.

Try to have your evening meal no later than 8.30pm and organize your evenings so that time after 8pm is all for you. Cooking a simple meal and savouring it should help you to relax and unwind. Include plenty of the Top 20 Anti-ageing Foods and make this meal higher in carbs than lunch. This will help you to wind your brain down towards bedtime.

Drinks Have at least 6–8 glasses of water or equivalent each day to keep yourself hydrated properly. See Food and Detox (pages 48–53) and Food for Your Looks (pages 24–31).

eating for health
A general healthy diet – high in fresh fruits and veg, grains, lean protein, nuts, seeds and pulses – is recommended in the 40s as for any age, but pay particular attention to foods that provide you with sustained energy (see the Glycaemic Index, pages 38) and most meet your particular health needs. Check the box on the left for food tips for health problems typical at this age.

treats to savour
Don't feel that you have to give up all your favourite edible treats or drinks to get your healthy diet. A glass or two of good-quality wine can be an excellent idea, too – but leave it at one or two glasses for optimum health and well-being benefits. (See the feature on alcohol and drugs in Well-being for Your New Life, pages 196–7.) In moderation, beer is an excellent drink in the evening, as hops are a sedative. Choose organic wine or beer to minimize the chance of a hangover and unwanted residues.

Chocolate can be very good for you because of its high antioxidant content – choose dark chocolate as it is higher in the beneficial cocoa solids. Tea and coffee are also rich in antioxidants and other plant chemicals that help protect against heart disease, while moderate amounts of coffee can increase alertness and concentration. Avoid caffeine-rich drinks with meals as it reduces absorption of vital minerals, like calcium and iron, and limit coffee intake to 4 cups a day.

> **If you suffer from ...** ibs **... try** honey, fresh herbs, fish, fruit, vegetables.
>
> **If you suffer from ...** headaches and migraine **... try** avoiding caffeine, hard cheese, alcohol – **and drink 6–8 glasses of water a day.**
>
> **If you suffer from ...** stress **... try** milk, turkey, camomile tea, chocolate, complex carbs.
>
> **If you suffer from ...** pms **... try** avoiding caffeine, alcohol and simple carbohydrates, and drink plenty of fluids. **Eat foods rich in vitamin B, such as whole grains.**

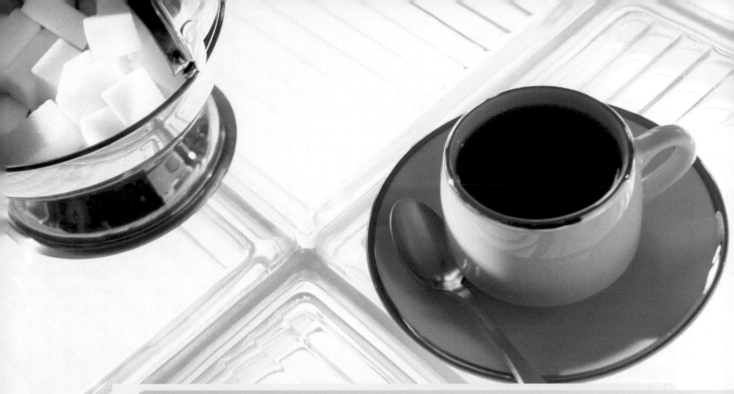

foods to avoid

sugar The theory that sugar gives you energy is faulty – sugar contains calories, which are converted to energy in the body, but all food contains calories. Sugary items can give you a quick energy fix, but if you want sustaining energy to last for several hours, they are best avoided. They cause your blood sugar levels to rise quickly and then, as insulin floods the system to cope with this sugar, you may feel weak, light-headed or tired.

For women before a period, this effect is heightened. Avoid snacking on sugary foods alone (and this includes fruit) when you feel hungry and/or tired as you will simply compound the problem. Instead, go for the snacks mentioned in How to Eat on the left, or a small piece of wholemeal pitta with hummus, or a pot of natural fromage frais. Such snacks are low on the Glycaemic Index, which measures how quickly food is absorbed into the bloodstream, and will keep you feeling energetic for longer, as well as keeping hunger at bay. Many simple carbohydrates, such as white bread, have a similar effect to sugar in the body. (See Food and Weight, pages 36–47 for more information on the Glycaemic Index.)

alcohol during the day Most alcoholic drinks (even dry wine) contain a lot of sugar and have a similar effect on your blood sugar levels as sugary foods and refined carbohydrates. Avoid drinking alcohol during the day and stick to drinking a little with a meal in the evenings. Women who suffer from PMS should avoid alcohol altogether in the week before a period, as research shows that intake exacerbates symptoms.

high caffeine intake While a small amount of caffeine spread out regularly is fine, excessive intake of high-caffeine beverages, such as brewed coffee or so-called 'energy drinks', is not a good idea. These can place a strain on the adrenal system and can leave you feeling wiped out and jittery at the same time.

around 50

Eating preferences and habits may be entrenched by the age of 50, but not difficult to change if the need is there – and, as we get older, it is more important than ever to eat the foods that will help maintain health and ward off the signs of ageing.

For women, healthy diet and weight maintenance can minimize the less desirable effects of the menopause, including hot flushes and tiredness. For more, see Food and Weight, pages 36–47 and Food for the Menopause (pages 54–9).

Although peak bone strength is built in youth, much can be done to help maintain bone density and thus reduce your chances of getting problems related to osteoporosis as you get older (see the box below). Osteoporosis is not only potentially life-threatening, highly debilitating and the cause of most fractures in older people, but also unsightly, causing body shrinkage and postural changes – such as an exaggerated stoop that can add years to your real age.

At this time, much can also be done to help prevent the major killer diseases of later middle age and old age – cardiovascular disease and cancer. (See also Well-being for Your New Life, page 168.)

bone builders

- Diet high in calcium (dairy produce, green leafy vegetables)
- Diet high in essential fatty acids (omega-3s and omega-6s)
- Weight-bearing exercise
- Diet high in fruit, vegetables
- Diet high in magnesium (nuts, seeds, whole grains) and vitamin E (plant oils, nuts, seeds)

bone robbers

- Diet high in animal protein
- Diet high in salt and the phosphates found in fizzy drinks and many processed foods
- Excessive consumption of alcohol and caffeine, and smoking
- Maintaining too low a body weight over time

do

● Eat up to 9 portions of fruit and vegetables a day. The latest information from the US National Cancer Institute says that perhaps the recognized advice to eat '5 a day' is, in fact, too low. Men should eat 9 and women 7. See Top 20 Anti-ageing Foods, pages 20–23, for the type of fruits and vegetables that may be particularly beneficial.

● Eat plenty of whole-grain foods. As well as helping to prevent certain cancers and reduce the risk of heart disease, they are also rich in nutrients and improve digestive efficiency.

● Eat pulses – e.g. soya beans, chickpeas and lentils. The US government allows manufacturers of soya foods to make the claim that regular soya intake can help reduce high LDL blood cholesterol (the bad type), and all pulses are high in soluble fibre.

● Eat oily fish. Oily fish, such as salmon, herring or mackerel, can help to prevent blood clots, heart disease, cancers and arthritic pain.

● Eat garlic and onions – they contain a variety of compounds which both help to protect your circulatory health and can protect against cancer.

don't

● Eat too much high-fat animal food, such as shoulder of lamb, fatty cuts of beef, Cheddar or Stilton, or cream cheese, cream or butter.

● Eat too many foods containing high levels of trans fats – fats that have been commercially hardened for use in mass-market products, such as margarines, biscuits, cakes, pastries and pies. These fats, also called hydrogenated fats, appear to be even worse for heart and circulatory health than natural saturated fats.

● Eat too many calories – being obese is a strain on the heart and obesity is also linked with increased risk of some cancers.

Maintaining a reasonable weight will also help to prevent the onset of insulin resistance, a precursor of diabetes and Type-2 diabetes itself. Although it is often said that insulin resistance (when the body has to cope with too much sugar in the blood and its ability to produce sufficient insulin is blunted) is directly due to high sugar intake, in fact that is only partly true – a high intake of calories of any type over time (a surplus of which converts to glucose in the blood) is more likely to be the cause. If you eat moderate portions, think 'little and often' and get plenty of exercise, you are much less likely to suffer from either of these conditions.

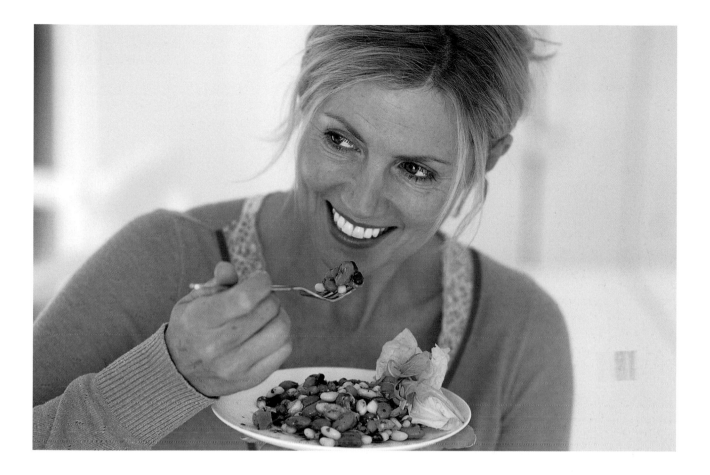

around 60

From early middle age your calorie needs decline steadily, so monitor portion sizes carefully to ensure you don't put on too much weight, which can be very ageing and can make you lethargic.

Research shows that older people tend to crave sweet foods more than younger people, so try to satisfy that craving with natural foods, such as fresh or dried fruits, rather than with a lot of cakes, biscuits or sweets. Choose top-quality honey rather than sugar, as it has healing properties. Try to keep your intake of salt reasonably low — high blood pressure is quite common as you get older, and sodium intake can raise blood pressure in susceptible people.

As liver function and digestion may become sluggish, many people feel happier eating smaller meals more frequently, so 2 mini-meals, 2 snacks and 1 small main meal may be ideal. Alcohol tolerance may also decline — but one glass a day is still good news for heart health.

A diet high in antioxidant vitamins, minerals and plant chemicals (see overleaf) will help protect you from disease and beat the signs of ageing. With a healthy diet you shouldn't need food supplements — however, co-enzyme Q10 can help maintain gum health and perhaps prevent the need for you ever to have false teeth! Fish oil supplements are an easy way to get your daily omega-3 oils with all their benefits (see Top 20 Anti-ageing Foods, pages 20–23).

Pain from arthritis and rheumatism can be minimized by eating ginger, chillies and fish oils, and the risk of stroke can be halved with a diet high in potassium (bananas and onions, for instance) and oily fish. Keep Alzheimer's and Parkinson's Disease at bay with a diet rich in oily fish (again!), nuts, seeds and olive oil, and maintain your eyesight by eating regular portions of carrots, mangoes and dark green vegetables.

A generally healthy diet, containing plenty of antioxidant foods, is also the best way to maintain your immune system in good order and help keep colds and 'flu at bay.

know your nutrients
During mid life it is vital that you get the optimum amount of all the 'micronutrients' that your body needs for good health and good functioning. Here we look at those nutrients, all needed in small but very important quantities, that can make all the difference to your health and well-being and how your body will age – and in the panel opposite we explain antioxidants and their vital role in holding back the ageing process.

what are micronutrients?

They are vitamins, minerals and phytochemicals (plant chemicals), and within this group I have also included essential fatty acids (special fats needed in small quantities, with a range of health benefits and anti-ageing qualities).

Vitamins are organic substances that are essential for a variety of roles in the body. The water-soluble vitamins are the B group (B2, B3, B6, B12 and folate) and C, and these should be eaten/taken every day as they cannot be stored in the body. The fat-soluble vitamins, which the body can store, are vitamins A, D, E and K.

Each vitamin has a different part to play in health, maintenance and well-being, and the amount and balance that we need depend, among other things, upon our age. Some vitamins, such as C and beta-carotene (sometimes called pro-vit-amin A, because the body can convert it into vita-min A) are also antioxidants (see opposite).

Vitamins B group and C are easily destroyed by storage, light and heat, so foods containing these vitamins should be bought fresh, stored carefully and given the minimum of cooking.

All vitamins are best taken as a natural part of food, as researchers believe that they can work synergistically with other compounds within foods. However, supplements can be useful on some occasions (see Section 4 on Well-being).

minerals
are inorganic substances, fifteen of which are essential in the human diet, either to build and maintain structure (e.g. calcium, magnesium), or to balance body fluids (e.g. sodium and potassium), or to regulate body functions (e.g. iron, calcium). Some of these are occasionally, or even quite commonly, in short supply in the diet, and poor diet and lifestyle factors can hinder their absorption or increase their excretion (this also applies to vitamins).

The best way to ensure adequate intake and absorption of vitamins and minerals is to eat a balanced, healthy diet containing a wide variety of meat, fish, poultry, eggs, dairy produce, pulses, whole grains, nuts, seeds, fruit and vegetables, and to lead a healthy lifestyle, avoiding excesses of alcohol, smoking, drugs, stress, etc. Different sections and features in this book will refer to various mineral and vitamin needs for different problems and occasions.

essential fatty acids
The essential fatty acids (EFAs, otherwise known as 'long-chain fatty acids') are part of the polyunsaturated family of fats. They are linoleic acid (the 'parent' fat of the omega-6 group) and alpha-linolenic acid (the 'parent' fat of the omega-3 group). Approximately 2g a day of both of these are needed for good health.

While the modern diet tends to favour the linoleic acid/omega-6 fats (found in many plant oils, such as sunflower, safflower, corn and sesame oil, and many modern processed foods), we may not get enough of the alpha-linolenic acid/omega-3 group, as they are found mainly in oily fish and in smaller amounts in dark leafy greens, flax seeds, rapeseed oil and some nuts and seeds.

The correct balance and amount of these essential fats is linked with protection from heart disease, strokes, cancers, arthritis, immune system deficiencies, brain health, skin health and much more. More on the EFAs appears in Section 4 on Well-being for Your New Life.

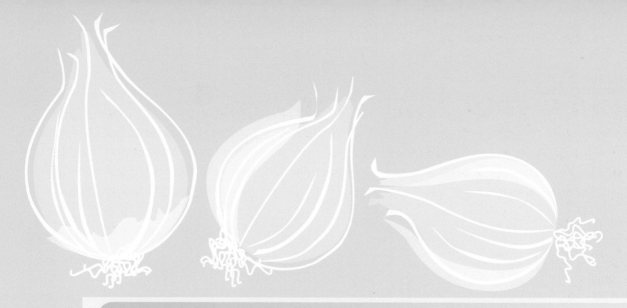

making sense of antioxidants

Oxidation is a chemical reaction that occurs all the time in the human body when human cells convert oxygen and nutrients into energy. Oxidation can be seen in action when metal turns rusty. This oxidation in the body produces particles called 'free radicals', natural by-products of everyday living.

However, when we age or are under stress or other negative lifestyle factors (for example pollution, smoking, drinking, illness), free-radical production is increased and it is thought that the physical signs of ageing, as well as the diseases of old age, such as CHD (coronary heart disease) and cancers, are directly related to DNA damage caused by oxidation.

Certain substances in what we eat and drink can counteract oxidation and are thus called antioxidants. Some vitamins and minerals, as well as a huge range of compounds in plants, have strong antioxidant properties. Scientists are now discovering that different types of antioxidants have different effects – for example, the compound in the spice turmeric called curcumin may be especially good at helping to prevent memory loss and Alzheimer's, while compounds called flavonoids, found in apples, onions and wine, are particularly good at giving protection to the heart, and glucosinolates, found in leafy greens, broccoli and cauliflower, can help to prevent cancers.

Some manufacturers have produced food supplement capsules containing particular antioxidants, but it is not yet certain that these supplements are as potent as the 'real thing' – proper food.

phytochemicals These are chemicals or compounds found in the plant foods that we eat (phyto = plant) which until recent years received little scientific attention but are now known to have important roles in health, anti-ageing and disease prevention. Many of these phytochemicals are antioxidants (see above), while others can act as natural hormone balancers, anti-inflammatories, painkillers, antibiotics and so on.

Fruits and vegetables are the main sources of phytochemicals in the diet, but whole grains, wine, beers and honey also contain beneficial plant compounds. So far, about 12,000 different chemicals have been found by scientists but new ones are being discovered all the time. A varied healthy diet including plenty of fresh produce is the simplest and best way to ensure that you get a good range of these powerful health allies.

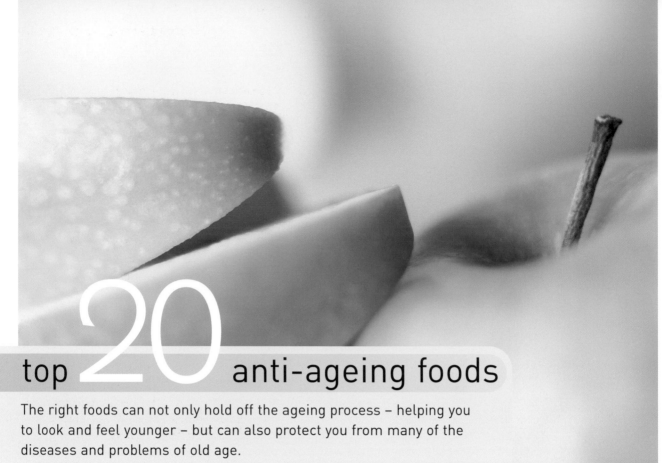

top 20 anti-ageing foods

The right foods can not only hold off the ageing process – helping you to look and feel younger – but can also protect you from many of the diseases and problems of old age.

These twenty foods are among the most important that you should eat on a regular basis.

apples

Apples are rich in two phytochemicals (plant compounds) called catechins and quercetin. Both these help to prevent strokes, heart disease and cancer. Quercetin has also been shown to improve the firmness of collagen, a component of skin that helps it to keep its elasticity and youthful appearance. Apples are also rich in the soluble fibre pectin, which helps to lower blood cholesterol. Lastly, the flesh of apples contains the mineral boron, which helps to prevent loss of calcium from the body and can thus help prevent osteoporosis.

avocados

Avocados contain an amino acid (the 'building blocks' of protein) called glutathione, which helps fight rheumatoid arthritis and Parkinson's Disease, and also protects against heart disease and cancer. They are

also rich in vitamin E, which is a powerful antioxidant (see page 19). Vitamin E is an important nutrient for good skin condition and protects against dryness and wrinkles, as well as helping wounds heal quickly and with minimal scarring. Lastly, they are a good source of monounsaturated fat, which is also linked to protection against heart disease (see Olive Oil).

barley

Whole-grain barley – sometimes called 'pot barley' – and other whole grains, such as rye and oats, contain a plant chemical called phytic acid which has been shown to inhibit the growth of cancers by its antioxidant and immune-boosting properties. Whole grains are also high in total fibre and soluble fibre, which helps keep the digestive and circulatory systems healthy and to prevent heart disease and diverticulitis. Barley is particularly rich

See also:
▶ The diet plans, pages 28–31;
▶ Making sense of antioxidants, page 19;
▶ Phytochemicals, page 19.

in chemicals called protease inhibitors, which also have properties that combat cancers, including breast and bowel cancer.

blackcurrants

Blackcurrants are one of the richest natural sources of vitamin C, at around 130mg per 100g when stewed. Vitamin C is an important anti-oxidant which protects against disease, helps to keep the immune system healthy, keeps the skin in good condition, and helps wounds and fractures to heal. High levels of vitamin C are linked with the lowest risk of heart disease. It is best to get your vitamin C in its natural form rather than via supplements, which may not have the same protective effects. Blackcurrants also contain other plant compounds such as lutein (see Greens) and anthocyanins (see Blueberries), and the oil from their seeds has been shown to have anti-inflammatory effects, relieving arthritic and rheumatic pain.

blueberries

Discovered in recent tests to be the most powerful antioxidants of all – 'mopping up' more free radicals than any other foods – blueberries have the strongest potential to prevent the negative effects of ageing and the diseases of old age. It has been found that 100g a day can stimulate the growth of new brain cells and may help prevent memory loss. Blueberries are also rich in a plant chemical group called anthocyanins, which help oxygenate the skin and carry maximum nutrients to the surface to help keep it looking young. Many other red, purple and blue berries have similar properties.

broccoli

Broccoli contains several important anti-ageing factors. It is high in antioxidant carotenoids, vitamin C and indoles, which help fight lung, breast and colon cancers. It is rich in lipoic acid, a fatty acid linked with increased brain power and energy. It is high in the

compounds lutein and zeaxanthin, which help keep vision healthy (see Greens) and is also rich in fibre, and is a natural source of chromium, which helps regulate blood sugars. It is higher in vitamin E than many other vegetables, and vitamin E is linked with protection against Alzheimer's Disease.

carrots

Carrots are richer than any other fruit or vegetable in carotenes – plant compounds which have a strong antioxidant effect that is important in helping to prevent cancers, particularly of the stomach and lungs. One study showed that carrot eating can cut the risk of lung cancer by half. Regular carrot intake can also help protect against macular degeneration and cataracts, can help minimize night blindness and can reduce blood LDL cholesterol (the 'bad' type). The carotenes in carrots also protect the skin from sun damage and skin cancers. Carrots should be eaten with a little oil or fat to help carotene absorption, and cooking them also helps.

celery

Valued across the world for years for its medicinal properties, celery is renowned for reducing blood pressure. This may be because of the plant chemical 3-n-butyl phthalid that it contains, as well as apigenin, one of the flavonoid plant chemicals. It is also an excellent source of potassium, a mineral that balances body fluids and can lower blood pressure in some. Celery also has anti-inflammatory properties and can help reduce pain from arthritis, as well as helping to beat fluid retention. One study found that celery is among the vegetables most strongly linked with protection from bowel cancer.

eggs

Good-quality eggs (i.e. those that are fresh, organically farmed and certified salmonella-free) are an excellent food, particularly as one gets older. They contain high levels of selenium – which may be lacking in the diet and has cancer- and heart disease-fighting qualities – and iodine, which can help to promote healthy thyroid hormone activity. An underactive thyroid can cause tiredness and weight gain. Eggs also contain lecithin, a fatty substance that can help to prevent heart disease and gallstones. Eggs are rich in a variety of vitamins and minerals, including vitamin E and zinc – both in shortfall in many older people's diets – as well as the B group, which helps nerve health and stress, and protein. Around 4 eggs a week are a good level to aim for (unless you have specifically been told to avoid cholesterol in your diet).

flax seeds

Flax seeds – sometimes called linseeds – are tiny golden seeds from the flax plant with several brilliant qualities. First, they are one of the few plant foods rich in the omega-3 fatty acid, alpha-linolenic acid, which converts in the body to EPA and DHA, two fatty acids found only in oily fish. These fats have a host of important anti-ageing properties – they help to prevent blood clots, stroke and heart disease, may help brain power and depression, can help arthritis and improve insulin sensitivity and are vital in retaining smooth skin. Flax seeds also contain lignans – oestrogen-like plant compounds that may reduce menopausal symptoms in some women.

garlic

Fresh garlic contains several compounds, the most important of which is allicin. Allicin has been shown to have potent powers to protect against several health problems, including high blood pressure, viral and bacterial infections, candida, indigestion, stomach ulcers and bowel disorders. Several studies have shown that it can reduce blood LDL cholesterol (the 'bad' type) by about 12%, and inhibits new growth of plaque in the arteries that can lead to heart attack or stroke.

Garlic may also help to prevent cancers by inhibiting the growth of cancer cells and strength-ening the immune system. Its high content of nitric oxide synthase may also help overcome male impotence. Onions, also from the same family, are rich in flavonoids and potassium, which can reduce blood pressure and keep the arteries healthy, and the onion family may also help to keep blood sugar levels even by regulating insulin production.

greens

Leafy dark green vegetables – such as Savoy cabbage, kale, and spring greens – are good sources of two carotenoids – lutein and xanthanin – which have been shown to help prevent age-related macular degeneration in the eyes, and cataracts, which are common in older people and can cause vision loss. Greens are also a good source of easily absorbed calcium to help maintain strong bones, while also being rich in potassium, which helps protect against calcium loss. Greens are also a good source of vitamins C and E, two strong antioxidants.

herbs

Several herbs are strong antioxidants even when used in the usual small amounts in cooking and salads. Thyme, oregano, rosemary, sage, basil and coriander all contain high levels of phytochemicals, which can help ward off heart disease and cancers. Oregano, for example, has forty times as many antioxidants as apples, according to the US Department of Agriculture, and in one study aged mice became more active when fed oil of thyme.

nuts

Nuts contain good amounts of magnesium, which is vital for energy levels. Magnesium can help maintain suppleness in the muscles, help avoid aches and pains, and may also help to prevent osteoporosis. Almonds, Brazils and peanuts are good for helping to build or maintain muscle mass and they can protect against glaucoma, Type-2 diabetes and high blood pressure. Research in the US has shown that just two 25g portions of fresh nuts a week reduced death from heart disease in male US doctors by up to 47%.

The fatty acids in nuts help to maintain soft, wrinkle-free skin as well as sexual function, and nut flesh is a particularly good source of vitamin E (see Avocados). Brazil nuts are rich in selenium, an antioxidant mineral that may reduce the risk of some age-related cancers and breast cancer.

oily fish

Oily fish, such as salmon, herring, mackerel and sardines, are the main source of the important fats called omega-3s (a branch of the polyunsaturated group of fats) in the diet. Such fish contain two particular omega-3 fats called EPA and DHA not found in any other foods. These special fats have been shown to have a wide variety of benefits to health, including protection against the decline of brain power and diseases of the brain, such as Alzheimer's and Parkinson's. They are also anti-inflammatory, helping to minimize the pain of arthritis and rheumatism. These oils can help all dry skin and allergic skin conditions. In addition they can help prevent blood clots, coronary disease and strokes. (See also Flax Seeds.)

olive oil

Although olive oil, like other plant oils, is almost 100% fat, it is rich in nutrients and compounds that can help protect against age-related disease. It is high in monounsaturated fats, which lower levels of the 'bad' LDL cholesterol in the blood while protecting the levels of 'good' HDL cholesterol, and thus protect against heart disease and stroke. Olive oil also contains the compounds squalene and oleuropein, which are powerful antioxidants, protecting blood cholesterol from oxidation. This antioxidant effect may also reduce the risk of some cancers, particularly of the breast and colon. Top-quality, cold-pressed olive oils are the best to buy for health as they contain greater amounts of the protective compounds.

onions

The onion family, including garlic and leeks, are good detoxifiers and are also antiseptic and antibacterial. Just 1g of onion a day is enough to help strengthen the bones, and the sulphur compounds contained in the onion family are also linked with protection against strokes, high blood pressure, heart disease and cancers.

spices

Most spices are strong antioxidants and have a variety of beneficial effects. Ginger is an anti-inflammatory and can help ease the pain of both forms of arthritis. Chillies speed up the metabolic rate, thus helping both weight control and circulatory problems. Chillies also contain the plant chemical capsaicin, which is a great reliever of general aches and pains. Turmeric has been shown to reduce the brain plaques which can cause Alzheimer's Disease, and coriander seeds can lower high blood pressure.

soya beans

Soya beans contain high levels of plant oestrogens and magnesium, both of which may help to minimize the symptoms of the menopause. Soya beans are high in soluble fibre, and have also been shown to help reduce the risk of heart disease. Soya protein helps build and maintain collagen and elastin, both important for maintaining skin in youthful condition. Lastly, soya contains good amounts of co-enzyme Q10, the compound that has been demonstrated to have a beneficial effect on both energy levels and gum health.

See also:
▶ Know your nutrients, page 18.

tomatoes

Tomatoes are rich in the carotenoid lycopene, which offers protection against cancer and heart disease. Recent trials have found that women who eat a lot of lycopene have a reduced chance of getting both ovarian and breast cancer, while in men it helps prevent prostate cancer. Lycopene may also help to protect against osteoporosis. Tomatoes are again a good source of lipoic acid, which helps increase energy levels and improve brain power in some people. Small – cherry or similar – ripe tomatoes tend to contain the highest levels of lycopene and cooking them helps their absorption.

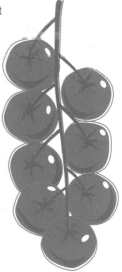

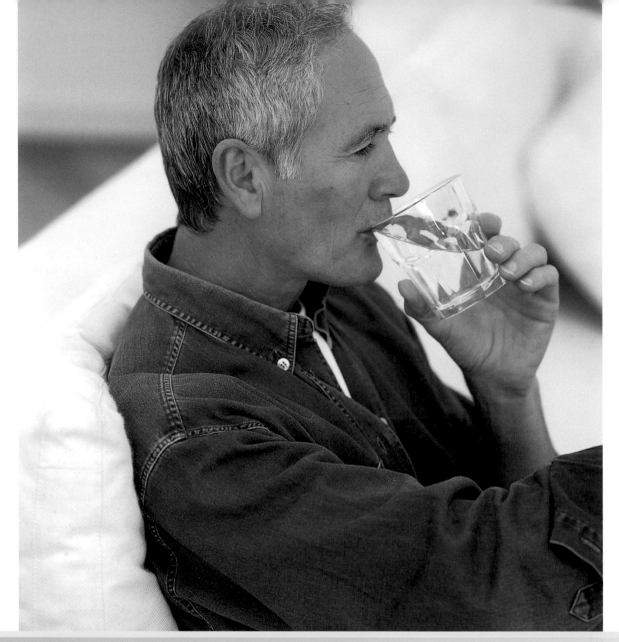

food for your **looks**

When the first signs of ageing show in your looks, don't automatically think of cosmetics, lotions, potions, creams, gels or drops as your main line of attack. If you want clear and smooth skin, shining hair, bright eyes and teeth and gums to make you smile, the best way to achieve these is to eat the right diet. At any age, beauty really does start from within. There are foods that can help moisturize and plump your skin, and protect it from wrinkles, dryness and sun damage; there are foods that will feed your hair and keep your eyes and mouth healthy – in fact there is a food, or nutrient, for virtually every problem connected with your appearance.

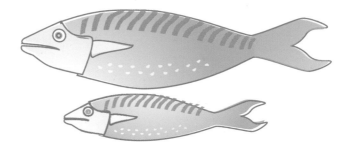

skin

The early signs of skin ageing include dryness and fine lines, both of which can be improved by simple dietary measures. Dryness is easily combated by a diet rich in unsaturated fats – particularly the longer-chain omega-6 essential fatty acids (e.g. evening primrose oil) and long-chain omega-3 fats (found mainly in oil fish). A daily supplement of both these oils should see improvement within two weeks. Relying on oily fish alone in the diet may not be enough, as (due to possible contaminants in the fish) the UK government says that we should limit ourselves to one portion a week, which would give only the equivalent of two day's supply of the omega-3 fats. NOTE: It is very important when eating a diet high in polyunsaturates also to eat plenty of antioxidant foods (see page 19) to ensure that these highly unsaturated fats, which are unstable, don't oxidize in your body.

Also remember to drink plenty of fluids as water literally helps to plump up the skin, avoiding that dried-prune look. In normal circumstances, 8 glasses a day would be about right.

It is also important to eat sufficient protein, which boosts the skin's collagen (to help plump up and pad out the outer layers of the skin) and elastin (which gives smoothness and elasticity). Lastly, to help avoid wrinkles and dryness, try to maintain a reasonable body weight and don't get too thin – a small layer of fat under the facial skin gives a smooth, healthy appearance, and often when people diet it is the face that loses the most weight.

A diet high in antioxidants (see page 19) is vital for good skin. It is thought that damage to the collagen in skin by free radicals is one of the causes of tough and leathery skin. Antioxidants are also thought to help prevent the appearance of age spots or 'liver spots' on the hands and other body skin. These brown spots, like large freckles, which eventually can meld into one large brown area, are thought to be a by-product of the oxidation of polyunsaturated fats in the body, which produces a surplus of a substance called lipofuscin. Antioxidants, such as vitamins C and E, and especially anthocyanins (found, for example, in blueberries and other dark berries), can help prevent this build-up if eaten regularly. Antioxidants will also help prevent the oxidation of long-chain fatty acids after you've eaten them (see page 18).

Some minerals are vital for skin health - for instance, zinc (found in good amounts in shellfish, whole grains, nuts and seeds) is vital for the manufacture of collagen and helps to speed up skin repair and renewal, and selenium (found in nuts, seeds, fish and offal) is an antioxidant mineral that helps counter dry skin and free-radical damage.

If your skin is frequently exposed to outdoor weather, especially in the summer/around snow or water or in the sun, you should eat plenty of foods rich in beta-carotene (one of the carotenoid group of antioxidants), such as carrots, mangoes, dark leafy greens, orange-fleshed melons and squashes, red peppers, broccoli and tomatoes. Regular adequate beta-carotene intake offers the type of protection from sunburn afforded by a low-factor sunscreen (although, if out in the sun, you should still use a suncream, of course).

Although long-term use of beta-carotene supplements isn't recommended, as very large doses have been linked with possible increased risk of cancer, short courses (say, starting two weeks before a sunshine holiday) of 30mg/day for a maximum of four weeks would increase your skin's immunity to the ageing and dangerous effects of UV rays. One study in 2002 showed also that supplementing with Vitamin C and E helps to guard against sunburn, although high doses of any vitamin supplement are not recommended by the UK Food Standards Agency. Lastly, there is some evidence that regular intake of foods containing the carotenoids lutein and zeaxanthin (see Eyes overleaf) may help to protect the skin in the sun.

thread veins – tiny, fine red veins that appear at or near the skin's surface, particularly on the face – are a common problem in the 40s and after. Sun damage is a common cause of the appearance of these, so do protect your face well from the sun, using a fake tan instead if necessary. There is also a genetic predisposition to inherit them, and pregnancy can make them worse. They appear more obvious when the skin thins as we age, so see tips above for maintaining collagen. Some people say that drinking alcohol and spicy foods makes thread veins worse, but I can find no proper evidence for this.

eyes

Sparkling, bright eyes can take years off your looks. Although other factors – such as lack of sleep, being over-worked or ill, or long hours on the computer – can make your eyes look tired and dull, a few changes in diet and lifestyle can improve them considerably.

Once again, a regular intake of the essential fatty acids (see Skin on the previous page) can help prevent some of the signs of eye ageing, such as dryness (a frequent problem as we get older), which can lead to irritation, a 'gritty' feeling, red eyes and more. Evening primrose oil, one of the long-chain omega-6 fats, may be particularly useful. You should also drink at least 2 litres of fluid a day to make sure that you are not dehydrated.

Dull eye whites can be encouraged to sparkle with a diet high in vitamin C, which will also help with redness. You also need to take regular outdoor exercise in the fresh air – it's surprising what a different this makes.

Red eyes and/or lids may be a sign of infection, so check this out with your doctor; otherwise it can be a sign of deficiency in vitamin B2 (found in yeast extract, offal, seeds, pulses and nuts) or zinc (shellfish, whole grains).

hair

Poor nutrition and high levels of stress are two common causes of hair problems in mid life, particularly of hair loss and thinning hair. If you find this a problem, increase your intake of iron-rich foods, such as lean red meat and leafy dark green vegetables, as well as of zinc, calcium, selenium and potassium.

You also need to take regular exercise to improve circulation. Hair loss in mid-life women is often caused by a decline in oestrogen levels, so it may be wise slightly to increase your intake of plant foods naturally high in oestrogenic compounds, such as soya and other pulses, yams and flax seeds.

Hair usually becomes drier as we get older, which can eventually lead to lack of shine and to brittleness – the hair doesn't look in good condition and can be hard to manage. Ensure that you have adequate fats in your diet (especially the omega fats already discussed), along with the vitamin B group and vitamin C.

Greying hair is influenced by genetic predisposition rather than by diet, but the greyer the hair the more it may look dry or dull, so follow the tips above to ensure it stays shiny and in good condition.

If stress is causing your hair to be in poor shape, see the tips on beating stress in Section 4 – Well-being.

teeth and gums

Good teeth are important at any age, but especially now. Your smile takes years off your face and you want to feel confident that people are looking at a gleaming smile and good gums. Apart from regular cleaning and flossing, and possibly dental care and or surgery, there is much you can do via diet to help your smile look better.

Avoid a diet high in sugars and sugary foods (even including fresh and dried fruits), particularly those used as snack foods between meals. Sugars left in contact with your teeth and gums for hours at a time will help to produce cavities, tartar and gum disease. Brush your teeth half an hour after any sugary food or drink. Note: Re fruit – we all need fresh fruit in our diets, so don't stop eating fruit, just remember to clean your teeth well afterwards.

Stained teeth aren't attractive, and stains seem to appear more readily as we age. Red wine and the tannins in tea are two major culprits in producing stains. If you like either or both of these (and both are healthy in reasonable quantities), use a stain-removing toothpaste.

Gum health is reliant not only on good hygiene but also on good diet. You need plenty of vitamin C (fresh fruit and vegetables) to prevent problems such as redness or bleeding, and a very useful supplement is co-enzyme Q10, which can achieve excellent results with problem gums after only a week or two of use.

hands and feet

For skin on the hands and feet, see Skin on the previous page. The hands are more prone to dryness than skin else-where on the body, probably because we put them in hot water and soap or detergent so much – and don't forget to wear protective gloves or use handcream afterwards. Nails, in particular, will suffer if they are dry, splitting, breaking and looking hard and unattractive.

The old wives' tale that gelatine is good for strengthening nails is NOT true. Nails consist mostly of protein, so a diet moderately high in protein is important to maintain their strength (lean meat, fish, dairy produce, nuts, pulses), concentrating on getting your weekly oily fish intake to help keep the nails supple.

If your nails are spoon-shaped (with a slight dip in the centre like the bowl of a fairly flat spoon), this indicates an iron deficiency, so increase intake of lean red meat, dark leafy greens and whole grains. White spots on the nails indicate a zinc deficiency, so eat regular portions of shellfish, whole grains, lean red meat and nuts and seeds. Nails take several months to grow from base to tip, so don't expect fast results.

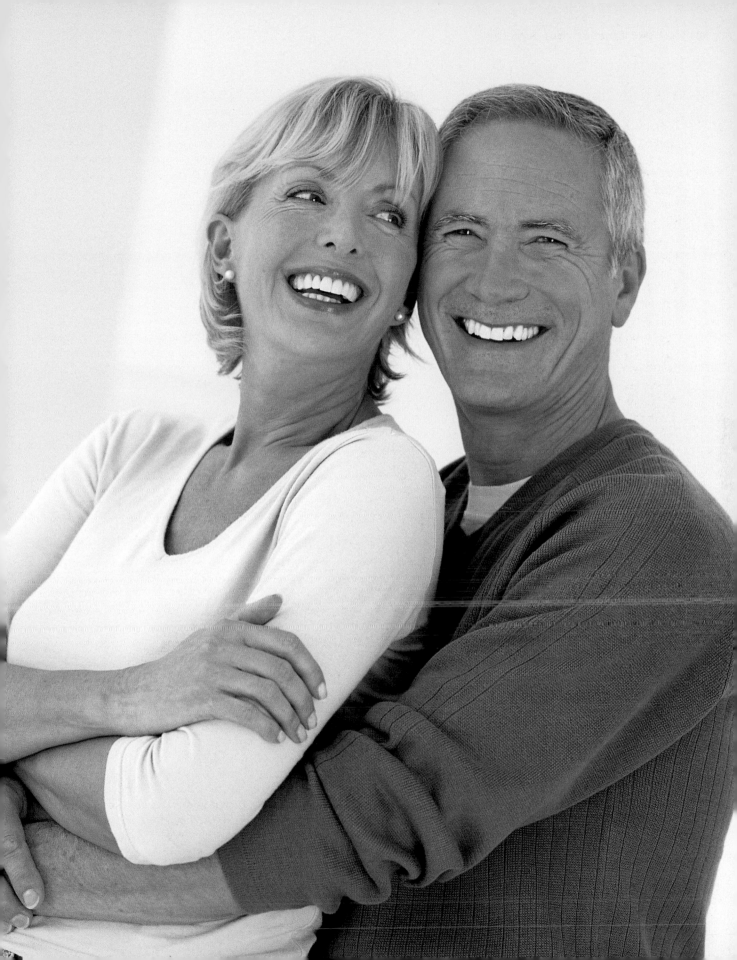

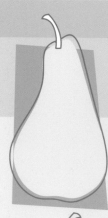

diet plan for your 40s

The plan here is suitable for anyone – both men and women – in good health, and will help to improve your energy, looks and ability to ward off the signs of ageing. Before beginning, check the list of tips below.

tips

● I haven't given exact amounts as you should adjust portions to suit your own appetite and needs.

● Add as much leafy greens and/or salad vegetables (raw) to the plans as you like.

● Drink 8 glasses of water or equivalent a day – some of this can be in the form of weakish green, black or white tea. You can have 3–4 cups of weakish coffee a day, but stop drinking coffee by mid-afternoon and don't count this towards your day's fluid intake (although coffee isn't as dehydrating as is sometimes claimed). Avoid tea and coffee with meals as they can hinder absorption of nutrients.

● It is better, nutritionally, to eat whole fruit rather than drink fruit juice, which is why there is no juice mentioned on this plan. However, the occasional real-fruit smoothie or breakfast glass of juice is fine. Vegetable juice is an excellent drink and doesn't contribute to tooth decay/enamel erosion.

● When choices are given, or a food is unspecified (e.g. 'portion of fresh fruit'), vary your choices as much as possible to improve your range of nutrient intake.

● Buy top-quality really fresh foods and take care with their cooking to preserve nutrients.

● If hungry between meals, snack on small handfuls of fresh seeds or nuts, or a small square of hard cheese.

day 1

breakfast
Fresh fruit salad
1 tablespoon sunflower seeds
1 teaspoon flax seeds
150ml low-fat bio yoghurt

lunch
Smoked mackerel fillet open sandwich on rye bread
Side salad of red lettuce, onions, tomatoes, watercress and olive oil French dressing
4 pieces of dried apricot

evening
Quick-fried sliced red peppers and beansprouts, with slices of lean beef fillet and broccoli florets, stirred in groundnut or olive oil
Wholewheat egg thread noodles
Compote of poached fruits in season
Low-fat natural fromage frais

day 2

breakfast
2 wholewheat biscuits, such as Weetabix, with semi-skimmed milk
1 orange
5 whole Brazil nuts

lunch
Crab and avocado salad with shredded Cos lettuce
Wholewheat bread with a little butter
Portion of fruit of choice

evening
Grilled chicken breast marinated in lemon juice and olive oil with thyme
New potatoes
Stir-fried shredded dark leafy greens
Carrots, steamed

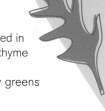

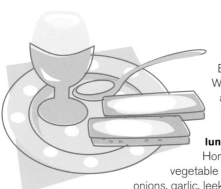

day 3

breakfast

Boiled free-range eggs
Wholewheat or rye bread with
a little low-fat spread
Pink grapefruit or fresh mango

lunch

Home-made or fresh chilled mixed
vegetable soup (including, for example,
onions, garlic, leeks, carrot, peas and spring greens)
1 tablespoon grated Parmesan cheese
Wholemeal pitta
Nectarine or plums

evening

Salmon fillet with good-quality basil pesto basted
over top and grilled until cooked
Brown basmati rice
Salad of mixed fresh herbs and mixed leaves,
dressed in olive oil French dressing
150ml low-fat bio yoghurt

day 4

breakfast

Whole-milk bio yoghurt with 80g fresh blueberries
and 1 handful luxury muesli stirred in
Whole-grain bread and yeast extract

lunch

Good-quality canned tuna in spring water, drained
and mixed into a salad with rocket, tomatoes,
wedges of Little Gem lettuce, sliced onions and
drained cannellini beans
Apple or pear

evening

Wholewheat pasta
Home-made tomato and basil sauce
Soft goats' cheese stirred through
Large green side salad

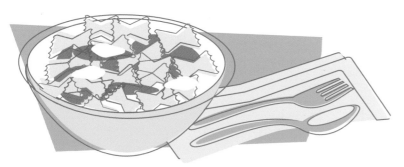

day 5

breakfast

Traditional porridge with good-quality honey and
raisins stirred in; semi-skimmed milk
Apple

lunch

Organic baked beans in tomato sauce
Rye bread, toasted, with butter
Orange or papaya

evening

Casserole with pot barley, sweet potatoes, onions,
cubed lean lamb
Steamed pak choi or spring cabbage
Low-fat bio yoghurt with honey

day 6

breakfast

200ml low-fat bio yoghurt topped with chopped
fresh fruit of choice, I dessertspoon each of pumpkin seeds and flax seeds and runny honey

lunch

Brie or Camembert cheese
Cherry tomato, rocket and onion salad
Rye bread
Apple

evening

Roast chicken (lean only) torn into bite-sized
pieces and stirred into a bulghur wheat salad with
chopped roast Mediterranean vegetables
(e.g. peppers, courgettes, red onion, aubergine)
Natural bio fromage frais

day 7

breakfast

As Day 1

lunch

Omelette filled with mixed chopped fresh herbs
(e.g. thyme, mint, rosemary, oregano, chervil)
Rye bread with low-fat spread
Grilled tomatoes sprinkled with olive oil

evening

Cod or other white fish of choice, baked
Sliced yellow peppers and red onion, stir-fried in
olive oil and garnished with coriander leaves
Baby new potatoes
Green beans

diet plan for your 50s

kick those bad eating habits Eating more healthily can seem like hard work if you've been on a less than perfect diet for years. Use these tips to help make the change easier:

● Make changes gradually – particularly about including more pulses and vegetables in your diet. This will help you to avoid digestive problems, such as increased wind or heartburn.

● Eat regularly. The meal suggestions in the plans here will help keep your blood sugar levels even so that you shouldn't feel hungry between meals.

● Don't be afraid to try new things.

● Cut down on sweet and salty flavours in your diet slowly. First cut out usage at the table, then reduce the amount you use in cooking and finally gradually give up high-salt, high-sugar foods such as crisps, salted snacks and sweets.

● There is no harm in small amounts of treat foods and drinks, such as wine or good-quality chocolate. Don't feel guilty about these, but try to have them with or straight after a meal.

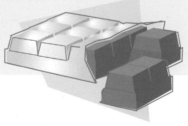

day 1

breakfast
Salad of red and black berries topped with natural bio yoghurt and sprinkled with sunflower seeds
Apple

lunch
Hard-boiled egg, sliced, with halved cherry tomatoes, sliced spring onions and fresh basil leaves served on dark rye bread and sprinkled with olive oil French dressing

evening
Sweet potato slices layered with spinach and topped with a cheese sauce made using skimmed milk, sprinkled with extra cheese and baked until cooked and golden
Broccoli

day 2

breakfast
Bowlful of luxury muesli with 2 teaspoons of flax seeds
Skimmed milk
Fruit of choice

lunch
Mackerel fillet in tomato sauce with a large mixed leaf and herb salad
Rye bread with low-fat spread
Red grapes or plums

evening
Griddled pork tenderloin
Steamed spring greens
Carrots
Mangetout
New potatoes

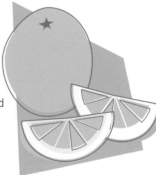

day 3

breakfast
Traditional porridge with runny honey and skimmed milk
Orange
5 almonds

lunch
Grated Cheddar cheese, onion and beetroot salad dressed in olive oil French dressing
Wholemeal or rye bread with low-fat spread
Strawberries or raspberries

evening
Poached undyed smoked haddock with poached egg on top
Spinach
New potatoes

day 4

breakfast
Low-fat bio yoghurt topped with any selection of red or purple fresh fruits
1 dessertspoon each sunflower seeds and pumpkin seeds
5 walnuts

lunch
Organic baked beans in tomato sauce
Baked potato
Grated cheese
Green salad

evening
Lean roast beef or grilled steak
Savoy cabbage
Roast butternut squash
Fruit of choice

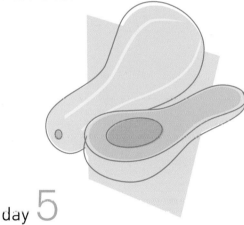

day 5

breakfast
Boiled egg
Wholemeal bread with low-fat spread
Pink grapefruit segments
5 Brazil nuts

lunch
Slice of salmon and broccoli quiche made with wholemeal flour
Large mixed salad containing a variety of leaves and herbs
Plums

evening
Chicken breast fillet stir-fried with fresh chopped chillies and ginger, pak choi and beansprouts in groundnut oil and a little light soy sauce
Brown basmati rice
Fruit of choice with low-fat bio yoghurt

day 6

breakfast
Special K with red berries
Natural fromage frais
Wholemeal bread with low-fat spread and good-quality honey
Red grapes

lunch
Leek and garlic soup
Wholemeal bread with butter
Parmesan cheese
Apple or orange

evening
Roast cod fillet
Green lentils cooked with onion and stock
Roast tomatoes with thyme

day 7

breakfast
As Day 1

lunch
Grilled goats' cheese
Rocket salad
Cherry tomatoes
Blueberries

evening
Casserole of chickpeas, squash, tomato, broccoli, and chicken thigh fillet
Spring greens
Wholewheat pasta shapes

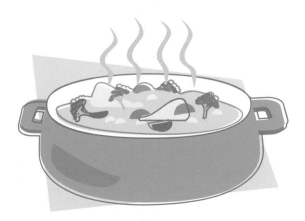

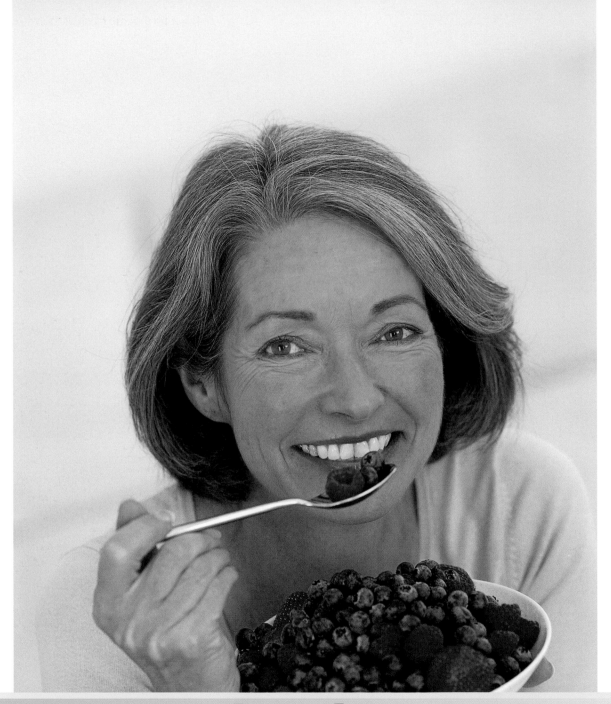

food for your **brain**

Brain power – including memory, concentration and speed of communication – tends normally to be at its peak in youth and young adulthood, and can show signs of decline in the mid years. Much can be done to stop this downward spiral, however, and the right diet is a very important factor.

There is plenty of evidence to show that if you want to maintain all your 'faculties' as you get older, there is no better time to begin making sure that you eat well than right now. Several types of nutrients have been shown to help maintain your brain in 'good working order' and prevent the brain diseases that most often attack in old age, including Alzheimer's and Parkinson's.

The first priority is to organize yourself a generally healthy diet, as outlined in the earlier parts of this section. For example, a diet low in fruit and vegetables and too high in saturated fat is strongly linked with a greatly increased risk of getting Alzheimer's Disease later in life. There is also a link between the type of diet that is good for maintaining heart health and one that is good for the brain, and people with high blood cholesterol and/or high blood pressure (two markers for increased risk of heart disease) are also at higher risk of Alzheimer's. It appears to be the antioxidants in a healthy diet (see page19) that have a particularly marked effect on reducing the risk of Alzheimer's. One large study reported in the Journal of the American Medical Association in 2002 showed that volunteers with a high intake of vitamin C, vitamin E, beta-carotene and dietary flavonoids were less likely to develop the disease.

Regular meals also predispose you to better brain power. There is much research to show that a good breakfast is important for brain function. A breakfast of whole-grain cereal and fruit has been found to improve memory by increasing your concentration, and the speed at which you process thoughts. This could be because breakfast gives you an all-important 'shot' of glucose after a long night's fast, and the brain relies on glucose for its energy. It could also be that breakfast cereals are rich in vitamin B group, especially vitamin B1, which has a special role in improving brain function.

brain food

The ancient belief that certain foods, notably fish, have extremely beneficial effects on the workings of the brain have recently not only received significant vindication from various scientific studies, but there seems to be a groundswell of public opinion in its favour. So much so that the supermarket chain Tesco announced in 2003 that sales of foods thought to be brain boosters were notably raised in areas with larger student populations such as Oxford and Cambridge. Sales of fish, broccoli, asparagus, spinach, bananas and all types of fresh fruit and vitamin supplements soared during exam time.

There is more on the power of fish for the brain in the later sections on Omega-3 fats and DMAE, and on broccoli and other vegetables (notably tomatoes) and fruits (notably blueberries), as well as turmeric and flax seeds, in the Top 20 Anti-ageing Foods on pages 20-3. We also look at brain-enhancing supplements overleaf.

Building on the foundation of a generally healthy diet and regular meals, all the following foods/nutrients have been shown to help improve brain functioning:

monounsaturated fats

During a 1999 Italian Study on Ageing, it was found that a diet that was rich in olive oil (which is very high in monoun-saturated fats) improved memory and helped prevent cognitive decline in old people, probably by maintaining the structure of the brain membranes. Monounsaturates are also to be found in good amounts in avocados and nuts.

omega-3 fats

There is much research to show that omega-3-rich oily fish really does prove the old saying that 'fish is good for the brain'. Fish such as salmon, herring, mackerel, tuna and sardines help to maintain the nerve function and the structure of brain cells, which contain a high concentration of these omega-3 fatty acids, and by helping the brain cells to communicate. The 'active' omega-3 oils in fish are called eicosapentaenoic acid (EPA) and docosahexaenoic acid (DHA) and they are found in no other types of food at all. One 1999 review of studies on DHA found that a diet rich in this fatty acid does indeed improve learning ability.

The action of these oils is helped if the overall diet is low in saturated fat. Also a diet that is high in antioxidants (page 19) will ensure that the omega-3 oils (which are part of the polyunsaturated group of fats) can work properly.

dimethlyamino-ethanol (DMAE)

All types of fish (not only oily) also contain a natural compound called dimethlyamino-ethanol (DMAE) which it is thought can improve your concentration and memory. Although there is little scientific evidence for its efficacy in this respect (for instance, the UK Alzheimer's Society advises members not take DMAE supplements) a diet rich in fish is worth a try.

vitamin E-rich foods

One 2002 study conducted by the US National Institute of Aging, published in the *Journal of the American Medical Association*, found that old people who had the highest intake of vitamin E were 67% less likely to develop Alzheimer's Disease, while a Japanese study showed that brain disease in mice could be halted by injections of vitamin E. A third study by Harvard Medical School, published in October 2002 by *Neurology*, found that a diet that was rich in vitamin E can lower the risk of Parkinson's Disease. In this study, over 124,000 people were followed for fourteen years. Vitamin E is to be found in olive oil and other plant oils, in avocados, nuts, seeds, egg yolks and various vegetables and grains.

vitamins B12 and folate

Low levels of these two B vitamins in the blood have been shown to increase the risk of Alzheimer's, according to a 2001 study published in the journal *Neurology*. Find vitamin B12 in lean meat, offal, fish, eggs and cheese, and folate in liver, pulses, fortified breakfast cereals and leafy green vegetables.

red wine

One large Danish study carried out over thirty years recently found that drinking red wine can lower the risk of getting Alzheimer's Disease by 50%. However, the amount of red wine needed is quite small – one drink a week is enough, according to the research! (see box opposite).

coffee

Drinking moderate amounts of coffee throughout life may improve your brain power, two studies have found. One (published in the *European Journal of Neurology*) found that three to four cups of coffee a day consumed since the age of 25 led to a 60% reduction in Alzheimer's Disease compared with people who drank 1 cup or less a day, while a study at the University of California found that elderly women who had been lifetime coffee drinkers outperformed non-coffee drinkers in eleven out of twelve tests of cognitive power. Interestingly, in this latter research trial, the coffee helped only the women – not the men. It is thought that this is because the ingredient in coffee held to be linked to improved brain power, caffeine, is processed in a different way in men and women.

supplements

Several supplements may improve brain power. Gingko biloba seems to increase capillary function and blood flow to the brain, which is an important factor in how the brain works (see also Exercise). Researchers at Tufts University in the US found that people with the highest blood levels of folic acid had little or no memory loss after middle age.

Supplementation with zinc and iron is also recommended by further US research which found that men given a low-zinc diet for three weeks lost their ability to quickly recall specific words, and women with borderline anaemia lost concentration and focus. Siberian ginseng may also affect the brain in a similarly positive way. The herb sage has also been used as a memory improver for many centuries, and sage tincture or pills can be tried.

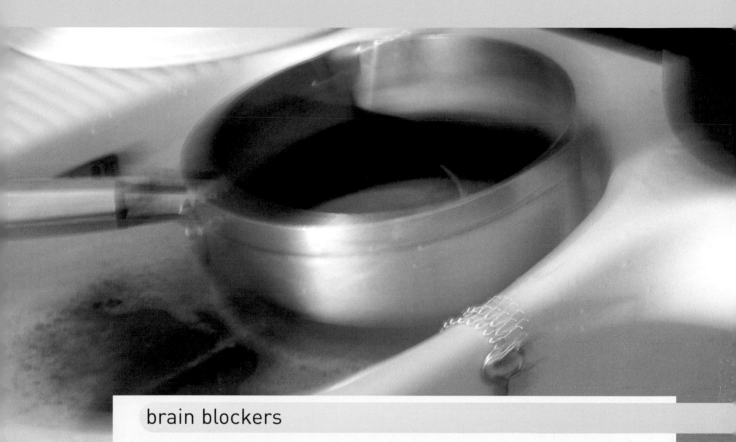

brain blockers

You can enhance the effect of the brain super-nutrients listed opposite by cutting back on certain items in your diet too.

sugar: Research conducted by the New York University School of Medicine has found that a diet high in sugar may encourage the hippocampus – the area of the brain that controls memory – to shrink. In tests, high blood sugar levels made participants perform badly in short-term memory tests. High blood sugar is also linked to insulin resistance (see page 16).

alcohol: Although small amounts of alcohol are good for health in older people in several ways, excess intake is not. Long-term high alcohol intake can affect short- and long-term memory – it appears to kill the brain cells.

saturated fats: A high intake of these blocks the work of the polyunsaturated fats (e.g. omega-3s), which are important for brain health.

In addition – make sure your diet doesn't include added aluminium!

There is some research to indicate that ingesting aluminium may be linked with memory loss and/or Alzheimer's, so don't use aluminium pots and pans to cook food, especially acidic foods such as fruits, as the aluminium can easily leach into the food.

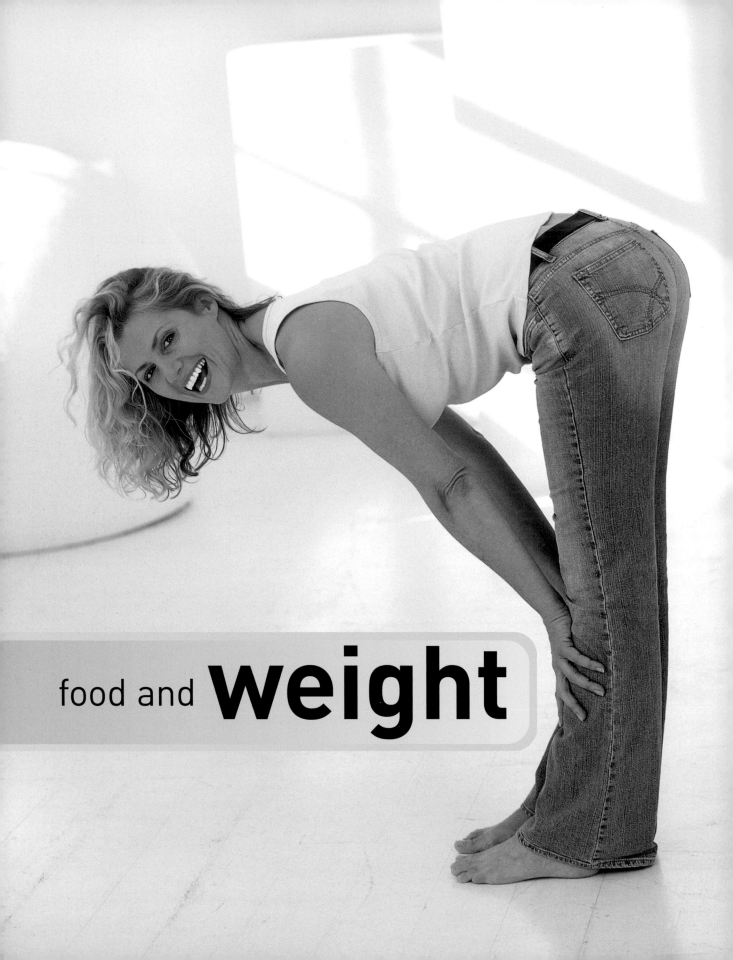

food and **weight**

Very few people reach mid life without having put on some weight. For many of us, this produces feelings of failure and guilt as we try to battle with the extra pounds – all too often, unsuccessfully. So here we examine all the middle-age weight dilemmas, sort out the truth from the fiction and provide tips and blueprints for easier weight loss without too many sacrifices.

It is estimated that 75% of people in England between the ages of 45 and 75 are overweight or obese, and, according to the International Obesity Task Force, the figures for the USA are similar, with an astonishing 40% of females from 45 to 65 actually obese (dangerously overweight).

If you are very overweight in your middle years, you are almost certain to be causing yourself health problems (if not now, then in the future) and may also be shortening your lifespan. According to one study published in the *American Journal of Epidemiology*, being overweight makes you around six 'actual years' older than you really are, and thus may shorten your life by a similar amount, while the UK Cancer Research UK puts the figure at seven years off an obese person's life, and the 2001 UK National Audit Office (NAO) report 'Tackling Obesity in England' said that deaths linked to obesity shorten life by an average of NINE years.

the facts are these:

● Obesity is linked with a wide range of diseases and symptoms which are most common in people over 40. Heart disease, stroke, high blood pressure, some cancers, insulin resistance, diabetes type-2 and osteoarthritis are the major ones, and it is now thought that overweight people are more prone to Alzheimer's Disease. See the panel on page 39 for more detail on obesity/health links. The NAO says that 18 million sick days, 30,000 deaths and 40,000 lost years of working life are caused by obesity in England alone.

● Obesity is also responsible for a range of other problems, including social isolation, depression and lack of self-esteem.

● Obesity is an increasing epidemic that has been put on a level with smoking as a cause of medical expenditure in the USA, and some estimates say that by the year 2020 most adults in the UK and USA will be overweight or obese unless something is done.

Thus, if you want to lead a healthy life in mid life, and stay alive for your allotted span, you should tackle weight problems now rather than later. All the research shows that it IS possible to lose weight in middle age – and keep it off. And it is never too late to do so. Even as the pounds begin to come off, problems such as high blood pressure, type-2 diabetes and angina may reduce in severity. And even if you are not severely overweight, keeping an eye on your calorie intake and lifestyle habits may prevent obesity in later years.

weight and good sense

Before you begin to try to shed pounds, you need to know if you really are overweight, for while obesity is linked with curtailed life, being too thin in your middle years is nearly as bad. That is because very low body weight is linked with greater risk of osteoporosis and low calorie intake can also be linked with a low intake of vital nutrients. Being too thin also predisposes you to dry skin and a greater chance of looking 'wrinkly'!

First check your Body Mass Index. Find out your current weight (without clothes) in kilograms (to convert pounds to kilograms, divide by 2.2). Now convert your height in inches to metres (multiply by 0.025). Then square your height (i.e. multiply your height in metres by itself). Now divide your weight in kilos by your squared height, and the result is your BMI.

If it is 25 or under, you are not overweight. (If it is under 22 in mid life, you are bordering on thin.) If it is between 26 and 29, you are classed as 'overweight', but for older mid-life people, a BMI of 26–27 is not considered of great concern. A BMI of over 30 is classed as 'obese' and this is when the links with poor health and shorter lifespan really kick in.

You should also consider your shape. It is better to be a 'pear' than an 'apple', whichever sex you are. Fat stored around stomach/waist is linked with greater risk of heart disease, syndrome X (opposite) and diabetes than fat on hips and thighs. A waist over 37 inches (92.5cm) for men, or 31½ inches (78.5 cm) for women indicates a slightly increased risk, while over 40 inches (1 metre) for men and 34½ inches (86cm) for women indicates substantially increased risk. After menopause, women are more prone to develop an apple shape, due to the reduction in female hormones, making the shape more 'male'.

the way to lose ...

If you do need to lose weight, you need to balance your food and drink (calorie) intake with the energy your body uses up. That normally involves eating and drinking a little less (of certain foods, see later) and taking a little more exercise on a regular basis (for more information on exercise and weight reduction/control, see pages 80–85). In mid life, even more than in your teens, 20s or 30s, you need to achieve this balance by eating healthily and by avoiding fad or crash diets. Although it IS a longer affair to lose weight as you get older (see Myths, pages 40–41), the weight is definitely easier to control in the long term if you do things sensibly and make changes in your eating habits that you can stick with for the next twenty years or so.

wise dieting

● As much as possible, choose foods that are natural and healthy. It has been shown that diets that are regularly high in items such as baked goods, confectionery, desserts, crisps, fast food and highly processed foods of all kinds predispose you to weight gain and make it hard to lose weight.

● Don't reduce food intake too low. Eating just 100 calories a day less over a year would result in a loss of 10 pounds. Studies show weight lost slowly is less likely to come back.

● Choose foods low or moderate on the Glycaemic Index. This measures how quickly foods are converted into glucose and absorbed into the blood. Foods high on the GI will be absorbed quickly and have you feeling hungry again before long, while low-GI foods keep blood sugar levels even and hunger at bay. A diet high in low-GI foods is especially important for diabetics and those with insulin resistance or syndrome X (see opposite).

Low-GI foods All pulses, whole-grain pasta, whole-grain rye, pot barley, pearl barley. Apples, dried apricots, peaches, cherries, grapefruit, plums, oranges, pears. Avocados, courgettes, spinach, peppers, onions, mushrooms, leafy greens, leeks, green beans, broad beans, sprouts, mangetout, broccoli, cauliflower, tomatoes. Yoghurt, milk, nuts.

High-GI foods Glucose, sugar, honey, pineapple, raisins, watermelon, ripe bananas. Baked/mashed potatoes, parsnips, cooked carrots, squash, swede. Brown/white rice other than basmati, rye crispbreads, wholemeal/white bread, rice cakes, couscous. Corn flakes, bran flakes, instant oat cereal, puffed cereal, wheat crackers, muffins, crumpets.

NOTE: The GI measures only carbohydrate foods, but both protein and fat foods reduce the rate of food absorption and so have a similar effect to low-GI foods.

● Choose a good balance of food types. A varied diet is important for health even while you are losing weight. Incorporate the healthy high-GI foods into meals which also contain low-GI foods, protein and a little fat.

● Eat 'little and often'. Research shows that most people stick better to weight-loss plans if eating frequently, with no more than 3 hours between meals or snacks. This doesn't encourage overeating, if meals/snacks are small and healthy. 'Little and often' has also been shown to reduce total calories eaten.

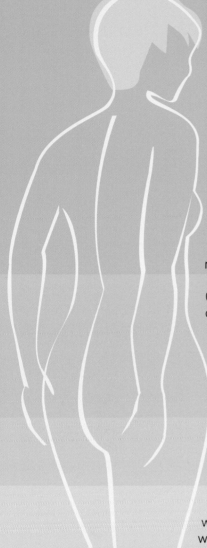

weight and health

Being overweight or obese in mid life is linked with several health problems. These are the main ones:

cardiovascular diseases
Excess weight, particularly around the midriff, is strongly linked with increased risk of heart and arterial disease and stroke, and of high blood pressure (hypertension) which can lead to cardiovascular disease. You need only be around 10% overweight to put yourself at higher risk of these problems. Abdominal fat is one of the five markers of insulin resistance syndrome (see below).

diabetes
Type-2 (non-insulin-dependent) diabetes, which used to be called 'mid-life onset diabetes' because it becomes apparent most often in middle-aged people, has overweight as its main risk factor. Research shows that woman aged 35–55 have a forty times greater risk of type-2 diabetes if they are overweight, and it is believed that approximately 75% of cases of diabetes could be prevented by maintaining a reasonable weight with a BMI no more than 25. Overweight can also lead to insulin resistance, which is often a precursor of diabetes.

osteoarthritis
This is a very common complication of obesity and it is believed that the extra weight causes undue strain on the knee and hip joints and the back.

cancer
Obesity increases the risk of colon cancer by six times, while in women it increases the risk of breast cancer. One large study found that there was a 100% increased risk in women in their 50s, probably because the amount of the sex hormones oestrogen and testosterone in the body are greater in obesity. Another study found that overweight increased the breast cancer risk by 40% in women aged 30–50, while overweight men increase their risk of prostate cancer by 20%. Cancer Research UK believes that one-eighth of all non-smoking-related cancers may be caused by weight problems, and the fatter you are, the greater the risks.

syndrome X
Also called insulin resistance syndrome or metabolic syndrome, IRS is officially recognized as a medical condition in the USA and someone is defined as having the condition if he or she meets at least three out of five criteria: central fat distribution (fat mainly concentrated around the abdominal area); high triglycerides (dangerous fats) in the bloodstream; low levels of the 'good' HDL cholesterol in the bloodstream; high blood pressure; and high levels of glucose in the blood. Reducing weight and taking more exercise nearly always improve all these five symptoms.

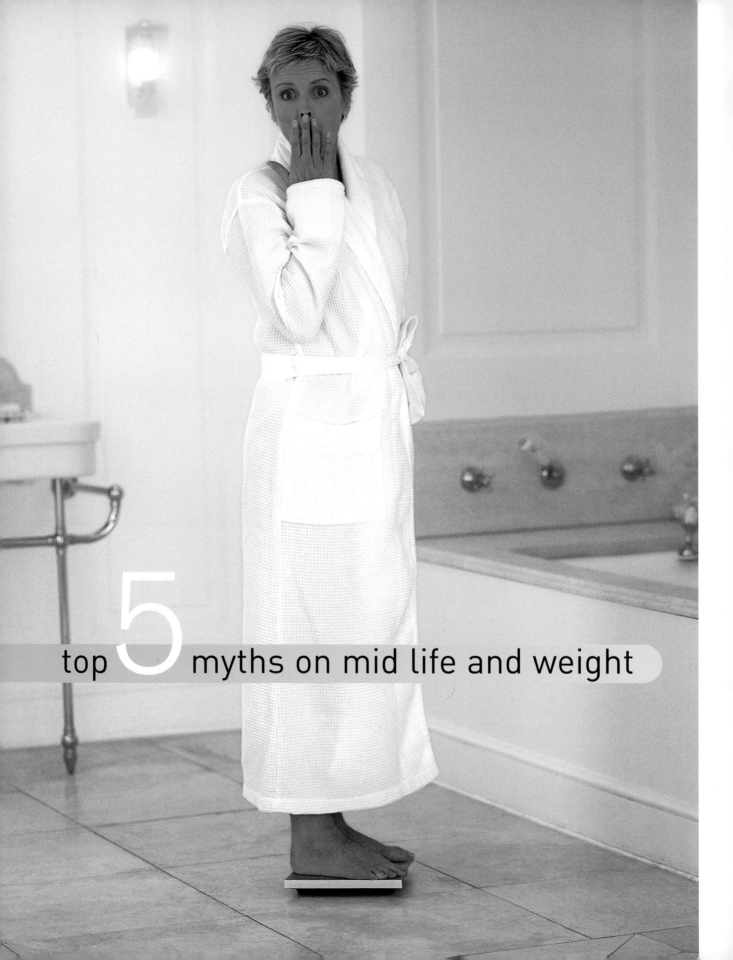

top 5 myths on mid life and weight

- **'It's my thyroid, doctor.'** Although a small percentage of people do have problems connected with the thyroid gland (its main job is to regulate the body's metabolic system) which predispose them to put on weight, most of us don't. It is estimated that 1–2% of people suffer from the medical condition hypothyroidism, symptoms of which can include weight gain, sensitivity to cold, tiredness, facial puffiness and swelling of the thyroid in the neck. Diagnosis can be made by blood test, and treatment is usually with synthetic thyroid hormone.

  However, up to 10% of the population may have some symptoms of a sluggish thyroid without actual full-blown hypothyroidism, which might result in a borderline blood test. Females are more likely to have thyroid problems than men, and early middle age is a typical time when problems may become apparent. For the 90% of people whose thyroid is fine but they are overweight – look to lifestyle factors as the likely cause.

- **'I'm fat so my metabolism has slowed down'** People who are overweight often blame a slow metabolism for inability to lose weight, which is quite the reverse of the truth. All research shows that the fatter you are, the higher your metabolic rate. This is, quite simply, because the greater your body weight, the more work your body has to do to carry itself around and do everyday tasks. If you then lose weight, your metabolic rate will slow down as you diet. This is one reason people find it hard to keep lost weight off. But research also shows that a previously fat, 10-stone person has a similar metabolic rate as an always-slim 10-stone person. In other words, dieting doesn't slow your metabolism per se – it is your new, lighter weight that is the culprit. If you want to stay slim, you will always have to eat less/exercise more than you did when you were fat.

- **'Middle-age spread is unavoidable.'** Although the National Audit Survey of 2001 showed that most people do gradually put on weight throughout the middle years, gaining on average 2 pounds a year, it is by no means inevitable. The main cause of this gain is that people tend to be less active as they get older, so that they burn up fewer calories in everyday life. Also, the proportion of lean tissue (muscle) – which naturally burns up more calories than other body tissue – diminishes. You can lose up to 5 pounds of muscle each decade after the age of 30 which, it is estimated, results in your needing about 100 calories a day less for every decade after that time; i.e., by the time you are 60 you will need 300 calories a day less than you did at 30.

  Both these causes of middle-age spread are largely preventable – keep active every day, and do weight-bearing exercise to maintain your lean tissue. These are discussed in detail in Section 2. Weight gain in the menopause is discussed on page 55.

- **'Yo-yo dieting over the years has ruined my ability to lose weight.'** Yo-yo dieting (constantly losing weight then putting it back on again) can mess up the metabolism, up to a point, by repeatedly diminishing the body of lean tissue (muscle). When you diet, some of the weight you lose (about 15%) is muscle not fat. When you regain weight, unless you do a lot of exercise, the regained weight is more likely to be fat than muscle, then when you diet again, more muscle is lost, and if this pattern is repeated over the years, by mid life a yo-yo dieter may have much less metabolically active lean tissue than someone who has never dieted.

  However, if you begin exercising, particularly weight-bearing exercise, research shows that you CAN replace lean tissue if you are determined, and that you CAN become a reasonable weight and maintain that weight. Time and patience are the keys – your motto should be, 'never yo-yo diet'.

- **'It's healthy to be plump in middle age.'** There is plump and plump. At 50, for example, it is probably wise to settle for a slightly higher weight than when you were, say, 25. This is because, firstly, being too thin can raise the risk of osteoporosis and can affect your hormones. To stay thin, most people eat a diet very low in fat, and this may make your skin, hair, etc. dry out – not a good side-effect if you value your looks. Fat has also been called 'nature's HRT', helping to keep oestrogen levels up during and after the menopause.

  However, a BMI over 26 or 27 is not healthy in middle age, so use your common sense. There is some evidence that fluctuating weight (e.g. if you are a yo-yo dieter) is even less healthy than being overweight – so go for a sensible weight that you can maintain without too much difficulty.

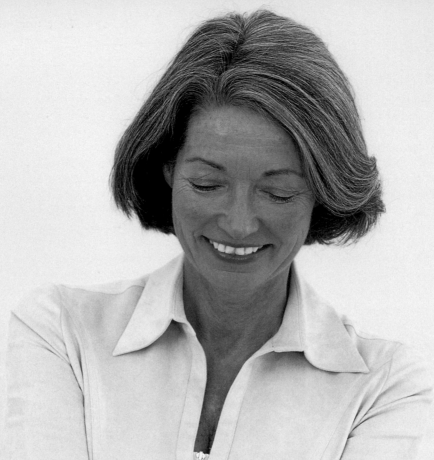

Somewhere between 40 and 60, strange things sometimes happen to your body. You may not be particularly overweight, but parts of your previously fine anatomy gradually begin to let the rest of you down. The most common causes for complaint that I've come across are the appearance of cellulite and a stomach that refuses to stay in line with the rest of your profile. Both these problems seem to affect women more than men, although men aren't immune. Here we look at the causes, and at what can be done via diet to improve the situation.

cellulite and troublesome tummies

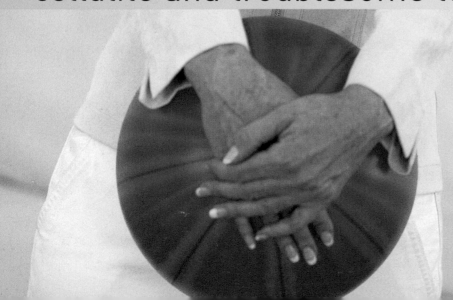

cellulite

The word 'cellulite' is a lay description for layers of body fat that congregate just under the skin, most often around the hips and thighs of women, and which have a dimpled appearance. This fat is chemically the same as other body fat, but the cause of the dimpling seems to be that, in women, fat cells under the skin are grouped in sacs held in place with fibrous strands of connective tissue, which doesn't expand even when the sacs are bursting with fat – giving the 'orange peel' effect. In men, the connective tissue is differently formed; most men tend not to lay fat down on the hips and thighs, and what is there is covered with a firmer layer of skin.

Cellulite may make its first appearance on your body as you head towards mid life and may take less exercise, put on a few pounds and the skin naturally begins to lose its firmness and elasticity.

What can be done? All research shows that most creams and potions on sale do little in themselves to cure cellulite. Indeed, the only treatments not related to diet or exercise that have been shown to have any effect are treatments with a powerful electric massager, called endermologie (available in salons only), and regular and vigorous massaging with a body brush, using any kind of lubricating cream.

There is also no proof whatsoever that a junk food diet, toxin-ridden diet, or any other particular diet, is the main cause of cellulite, unless such a diet causes you to put on weight, because even a few pounds overweight – if it tends to go to your lower body – may make cellulite dimples appear worse.

The best lines of attack are to stay slim and to take regular aerobic and strength training exercise (concentrating on the lower body). For more on cellulite and exercise, see page 73. You may like to use the Detox Diet on pages 52–3, but again, in itself, the diet has no special magic powers to get rid of cellulite and the weight- loss plans that follow are a good starting point, although you shouldn't expect fast results. It may take several months.

tummy troubles

The main dietary cause of a stomach that seems to have a life of its own is bloating. This is usually due to fluid retention or gasses, and both problems can largely be corrected by diet (thank goodness!).

Fluid retention is usually caused by a diet high in carbohydrates, particularly refined white carbs, such as white bread, cakes, biscuits and pasta, but also by sugar and sugary foods. These attract water as they pass through the system, and cause a lot of extra fluid to be retained (often around the stomach). As soon as you cut back on such items you will go to the loo more frequently and your stomach will shrink.

Another cause of fluid retention is a high-salt diet, so you need to cut back on salty foods like crisps (double whammie these, as they are also a high-carb food) and savoury snacks, and junk and processed foods of all kinds. Eating a diet rich in potassium helps eliminate fluid from the body – eat plenty of fresh fruit and veg. Other diuretic foods include many fresh herbs (parsley particularly) and salad vegetables, such as celery, and watermelons.

If bloating is due to gasses in the lower intestine, then try to find out what causes you to produce too much gas. Common triggers are pulses, cabbage, onions, dried fruits, dairy produce, wheat, yeast, coffee and alcohol. Eliminate these one by one, as you don't want to give up healthy foods such as pulses or onions unless you have to. TIP: If pulses or veg cause your bloating, cooking thoroughly and puréeing (in a soup or casserole) can often effect a cure. Also eat 'little and often' if prone to bloating caused by fluid retention OR gas. The Detox Diet on pages 52–3 should help with bloating as it incorporates all the dietary tips here. For more information on bloating, see Irritable Bowel Syndrome, page 192. **NOTE:** A large stomach can also be caused by intra-abdominal fat, which can be caused by stress, menopause or a genetic tendency to apple shape.

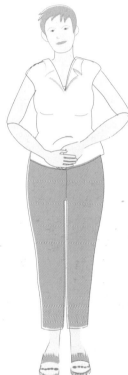

eat fat! Very-low-fat diets are linked with depression, dry skin, and a range of health problems. Make sure to include some oily fish (for omega-3s), nuts and seeds (for omega-6s), avocado and olive oil (for monounsaturates) in your diet on a regular basis. Small amounts of natural saturates (e.g. in butter, meat and dairy produce) are also fine and help you to feel satisfied after a meal. Moderation is the key.

diets for weight loss

plan 1 For women and men with under 1 stone to lose

● This plan provides about 1,500 calories/day, which will result in steady weight loss for most women and for men with under 1 stone to lose, as long as it is combined with regular exercise (see Section 2).

● Every day you have an allowance of 250ml skimmed milk for use in tea and coffee (up to 4 cups) or as a drink on its own. If you don't want this, have 200ml low-fat bio yoghurt instead.

● You can also have unlimited green salad items and leafy green veg, such as lettuce, rocket, cucumber, spring greens, red cabbage.

● Unlimited are any fat-free salad dressings, herbs, spices, vinegars, lemon juice, soya sauce or Worcestershire sauce.

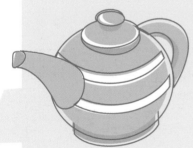

● You can have unlimited water, tea and herbal tea.

● Every day you can have a medium glass of dry white or red wine or champagne. If you don't want this you can have a small chocolate wafer bar or any treat to 100 calories.

monday

breakfast
2 wholewheat biscuits, such as Weetabix, with skimmed milk (extra to allowance)
1 peach or 2 plums
5 whole almonds and 5 walnut halves

snack
1 apple

lunch
1 medium breakfast bowlful of couscous (reconstituted according to pack instructions) tossed with 100g cooked chickpeas, chopped red pepper, cucumber and spring onion, and 1 tablespoon olive oil French dressing.
1 low-fat fruit yoghurt, any flavour

snack
1 dark rye crispbread with l level dsp vegetable pâté

evening
6 king prawns OR 150g monkfish, cut into pieces, marinated in harissa paste and grilled
200g (cooked weight) brown basmati rice
Large side salad with oil-free French dressing

tuesday

breakfast
200ml low-fat bio yoghurt topped with 150g mixed chopped (as necessary) fresh fruit of choice
1 level tablespoon pumpkin seeds
1 dessertspoon runny honey

snack
Apple

lunch
Takeout tuna and salad sandwich on wholemeal bread
5 almonds
l medium banana

snack
100g natural fromage frais

evening
100g lean rump steak, sliced and stir-fried in 1 dessertspoon groundnut or olive oil with a 200g selection of mixed vegetables (e.g. mangetout, sweetcorn, carrot, broccoli), sliced thinly as necessary, finished with a dash of chilli sauce and light soy sauce
200g portion (cooked weight) whole-wheat egg thread noodles

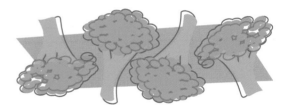

wednesday

breakfast
1 (40g) slice of whole-grain bread or toast with 2 teaspoons low-fat spread and honey
100ml fresh orange juice
100g pot of diet fruit yoghurt

snack
1 pear or 2 plums

lunch
1 ready-to-eat pasta salad, any selection, containing not more than 350 calories
1 medium banana

snack
Handful (15g) of sunflower seeds

evening
120g salmon steak, brushed with a little good-quality ready-made basil pesto and grilled until cooked through – about 4–5 minutes
150g new potatoes
100g green beans or broccoli
60g baby corn cobs

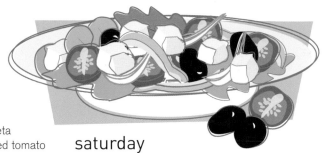

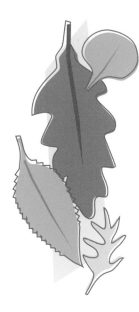

thursday

breakfast
As Tuesday

snack
2 dried ready-to-eat figs

lunch
Greek salad made using 75g crumbled Feta cheese, crisp salad leaves, roughly chopped tomato or halved cherry tomatoes, cucumber, spring or red onion, finely sliced red or yellow peppers, a few halved stoned black olives and 1 tablespoon olive oil French dressing
25g slice wholemeal or dark rye bread

snack
Apple

evening
75g (dry weight) pasta of choice, cooked according to pack instructions and tossed with 120ml good-quality ready-made tomato sauce for pasta
1 level tablespoon shaved Parmesan cheese
Large green side salad with oil-free dressing

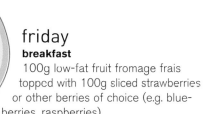

friday

breakfast
100g low-fat fruit fromage frais topped with 100g sliced strawberries or other berries of choice (e.g. blueberries, raspberries)
1 (25g) slice of whole-grain or dark rye bread with 1 teaspoon low-fat spread and honey

snack
5 whole almonds

lunch
50g dressed crab tossed with 1 tablespoon low-fat mayonnaise mixed with 1 tablespoon low-fat bio yoghurt and a little lime juice and rolled in 1 tortilla with chopped salad items of choice
1 slice of cantaloupe melon or 1 peach

snack
1 dark rye crispbread with 1 dessertspoon vegetable pâté

evening
175g chicken breast fillet, cut into bite-sized pieces, marinated in lemon juice with crushed garlic, ready-crushed chilli and fresh coriander leaves plus seasoning to taste, then threaded on a kebab skewer and grilled for 8 minutes, turning once, until cooked through
200g (cooked weight) brown basmati rice
Tomato and onion side salad with 1 tablespoon olive oil French dressing

saturday

breakfast
75g no-added-sugar-or-salt luxury muesli
Skimmed milk to cover (extra to allowance)
1 nectarine or pear

snack
5 walnut halves

lunch
1 carton of any chilled ready-to-eat vegetable soup (without added cream), containing no more than 200 calories per carton
1 small wholemeal roll with 1 teaspoon butter

snack
100g low-fat fromage frais

evening
200g portion of cod fillet topped with 2 tablespoons ready-made good-quality Mediterranean sauce for pasta and baked at 180°C/gas 4 for 20 minutes or until cooked through
150g new potatoes
75g petit pois
75g broccoli
1 small banana

sunday

breakfast
2 (25g) slices of extra-lean back bacon, grilled and served with 1 medium poached egg, 1 grilled tomato and 2 tablespoons low-sugar, low-salt baked beans in tomato sauce
1 (25g) slice of wholemeal bread with 1 teaspoon low-fat spread

lunch
150g roast chicken breast (no skin)
150g new potatoes
Steamed greens
Steamed carrots
Fat-skimmed gravy
150g mixed berries topped with 1 tablespoon Greek yoghurt and 1 teaspoon caster sugar

evening
Sandwich of 2 (25g) slices of wholemeal bread with 2 teaspoons low-fat spread, filled with 100g tuna in spring water, well drained, salad items of choice and 1 dessertspoon low-fat mayonnaise.
1 apple or orange

diet plan 2

For men with more than 1 stone to lose and women with more than 3 stones to lose
This plan is based on getting about 1,700 calories a day. The daily allowances etc. are the same as for Plan 1. If you find you are not losing weight at a rate of at least a pound per week on this diet, change to Plan 1.

monday
breakfast
1 (150ml) pot of low-fat bio yoghurt, any flavour, with 1 dessertspoon sunflower seeds sprinkled in it
1 medium banana
1 satsuma or kiwi fruit
snack
5 whole Brazil nuts
lunch
Avocado salad: mix 1 small sliced ripe avocado with mixed salad leaves, sliced red onion, halved cherry tomatoes and 1 level dessertspoon pine nuts, with 1 tablespoon olive oil French dressing
1 small wholemeal roll
snack
1 dark rye crispbread with 1 dessertspoon vegetable pâté
evening
1 (150g) lamb steak, grilled
200g (reconstituted weight) couscous
100g broccoli

tuesday
breakfast
1 (40g) slice of wholemeal bread, toasted and topped with 150g low-sugar, low-salt baked beans in tomato sauce
100ml fresh orange juice
snack
5 almonds
lunch
1 (250g) baked potato topped with 100g tuna in spring water, drained and mixed with 1 tablespoon low-fat mayonnaise and a little lemon juice and pepper
Large mixed side salad with 1 tablespoon olive oil French dressing
1 apple or pear
snack
100g pot of diet fromage frais
evening
Omelette made from 2 large eggs, cooked in a non-stick pan with 2 teaspoons groundnut oil, filled with a mixture of thinly sliced button mushrooms, fresh beansprouts and coriander leaves and a dash of light soy sauce
125g new potatoes, cooked and then chopped and sautéed in 2 teaspoons groundnut oil
100g petit pois
100g steamed pak choi

wednesday
breakfast
Milkshake: Blend 200ml semi-skimmed milk with l small peeled banana, roughly chopped, 100g sliced hulled strawberries and 2 teaspoons runny honey. Serve chilled
1 (25g) slice of wholemeal bread with 1 teaspoon low-fat spread and Marmite or reduced-sugar jam
snack
5 Brazil nuts
lunch
1 wholemeal pitta bread or wrap filled with 1 heaped tablespoon good-quality hummus, served with a selection of raw vegetables such as carrot, celery, peppers and tomato
1 apple
snack
100g low-fat fromage frais
evening
Chicken Caesar salad: Cook 1 (150g) chicken breast fillet and remove skin, slice and place on a large bowlful of torn Cos lettuce leaves dressed with a good-quality ready-made Caesar salad dressing; top with baked croutons
1 orange

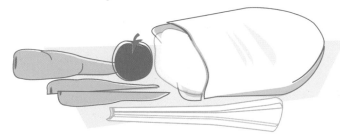

thursday

breakfast

75g luxury muesli with 1 level tablespoon sunflower seeds sprinkled over and with 1 apple chopped in Skimmed milk to cover (extra to allowance)

snack

1 dark rye crispbread with 2 teaspoons Marmite

lunch

1 (100g) smoked mackerel fillet
1 (25g) slice of wholemeal bread with 2 teaspoons low-fat spread
Large green side salad with oil-free dressing
1 medium banana

snack

Apple

evening

100g ball of mozzarella, thinly sliced and interleaved with 1 thinly sliced beef tomato in an individual gratin dish, with fresh basil leaves sprinkled over and 1 tablespoon olive oil French dressing plus a dash of balsamic vinegar; place under a hot grill for 2 minutes or until the cheese is partially melted and serve with 1 (40g) slice of crusty wholemeal bread to mop up the juices
1 satsuma or kiwi fruit

friday

breakfast

2 wholewheat biscuits, such as Weetabix, with skimmed milk (extra to allowance)
1 peach or nectarine
25g wholemeal bread with 1 teaspoon low-fat spread and runny honey

snack

Small handful of pumpkin seeds

lunch

2 (25g) slices of dark rye bread with 2 teaspoons low-fat spread, filled with 1 medium hard-boiled egg, sliced, 50g peeled prawns, 1 level dessertspoon low-fat mayonnaise and salad of choice
1 apple

snack

150g pot of low-fat bio yoghurt

evening

Vegetable curry: Cook 100g firm potato chunks and 100g butternut squash chunks until almost tender, then stir both in a non-stick pan with 2 teaspoons groundnut oil and 2 teaspoons good-quality ready-made curry paste of choice, then add 50ml ready-made chilled vegetable stock, 50g spinach leaves and 25g cooked green beans; cover and simmer for 20 minutes; stir in 25ml low-fat bio yoghurt and serve on 200g (cooked weight) basmati rice

saturday

breakfast

As Monday

snack

5 walnut halves

lunch

1 carton of any chilled ready-to-eat vegetable soup (without added cream), containing no more than 200 calories per carton
1 small wholemeal roll with 1 teaspoon butter

snack

4 dried ready-to-eat apricot pieces

evening

1 whole medium trout, grilled until cooked through
25g flaked toasted almonds
150g new potatoes
100g green beans
60g sweetcorn kernels or peas
Lemon wedge, to garnish

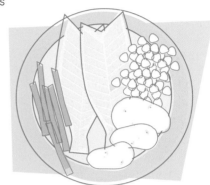

sunday

breakfast

2 medium eggs, poached
1 (40g) slice of wholemeal bread, toasted with 2 teaspoons low-fat spread
100ml fresh orange juice

snack

5 walnut halves

lunch

3 traditional oatcakes
2 tablespoons good-quality ready-made guacamole
Tomato and red onion side salad with oil-free dressing

evening

150g lean roast beef OR trimmed steak, grilled
1 (200g) baked potato
Large portion of steamed greens
Steamed carrots
Fat-skimmed gravy
150ml portion of fresh fruit salad with 1 tablespoon Greek yoghurt

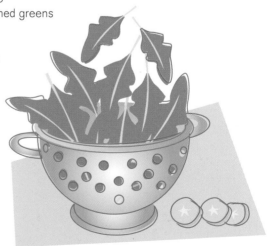

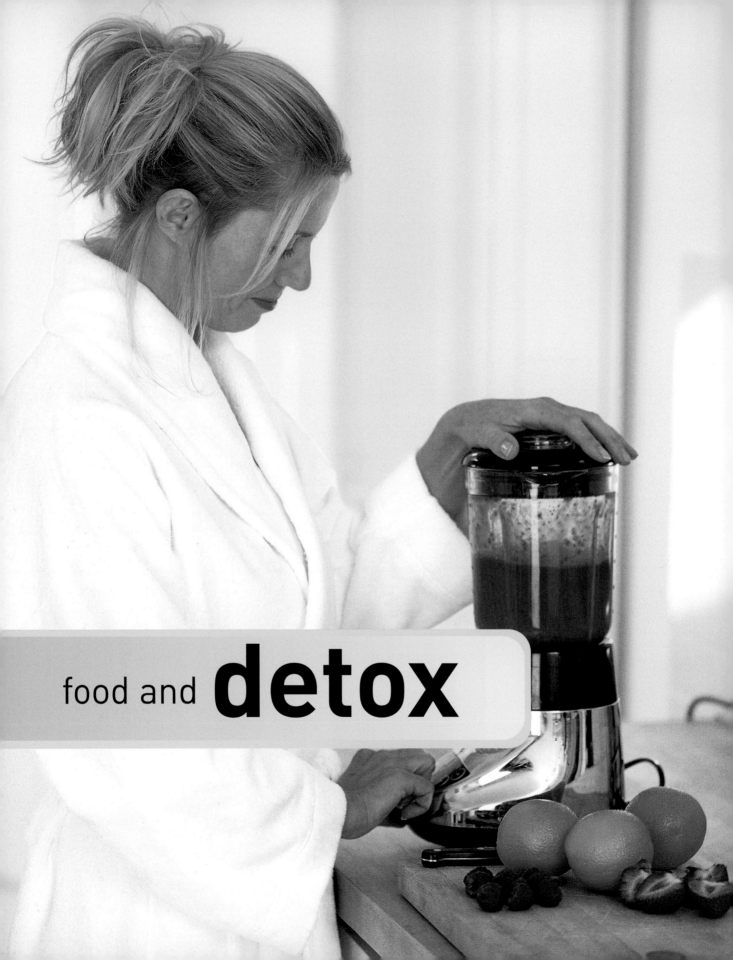

food and **detox**

If you're not exactly ill, but nevertheless feeling a bit under par – perhaps tired all the time, lethargic, lacking in your old sparkle or zest for life – you may have considered doing a 'detox' programme. After all, everyone else seems to have done it. Here we ask, is a detox really for you? And provide all the answers...

There's probably been more nonsense talked and written about the mysterious process of 'detoxing' than almost any other diet or health matter. Here are the answers to all your questions.

what is a detox? A detox is the process of ridding your body (and, some say, your mind, perhaps even your whole life) of negative and/or unnecessary baggage and/or pollutants that are creating unwanted effects. A dietary detox (what mainly concerns us here) generally takes the form of switching to a diet high in the foods and drinks that will actively promote a detox effect, while avoiding the foods and drinks which are negative in this respect. What exactly these diet items consist of is the subject of much debate among 'detox' experts.

does a detox diet work? It is certainly possible to feel better in several ways at the end of a detox – for instance, most people report feeling less tired and much less lethargic, with increased energy. Many report better skin and brighter eyes, and almost all tend to lose weight.

how does a detox work? There are many claims made for how and why detoxes work to make you feel better and look better, but most claims are based on the idea that chemicals in the chosen detox foods help purge your body of 'toxins', such as heavy metals, drug residues and other pollutants, and that the banned foods are those which, in one of several ways, may encourage toxicity in your body.

In truth, a good detox diet is simply a high-vitamin, high-antioxidant short-term diet which increases your fluid, fruit and vegetable intake and reduces the amount of highly processed foods that you eat. All detoxes require you to give up a long list of foods, the usual no-nos being those containing additives, residues, salt, added sugar, wheat and animal fat. The less healthy your pre-detox diet is, the more likely you are to feel better after the detox, but few of the individual foods on a detox have any particularly miraculous properties; it is a combination of factors that produces results. Indeed, many of the foods that are often banned – like bread, potatoes, meat and fish – are, or can be, perfectly healthy foods for most people. Their exclusion may be more a matter of opinion than science.

are there any negative side-effects of detoxing? In the short term, many people report headaches, probably due to withdrawal symptoms from caffeine, or even from a food to which you may be mildly intolerant (e.g. dairy produce or wheat). Others report a breakout of spots or blotchy skin, which could be due to a high intake of fruits or, as many detox experts claim, is an indication of the 'poisons' eliminating themselves from your body. Some people actually feel more tired in the first days of a detox. All these symptoms tend to disappear about 3–5 days into the detox.

when the detox is over, what should I do? Gradually begin including a little more food in your diet, adding portions of healthy foods that your detox has avoided – e.g. root vegetables, fish, poultry. If particular problems have cleared up on your detox – e.g., irritable bowel syndrome – then reintroduce foods one by one to see if you can find the culprit. For most people, however, a balanced diet, including a wide range of foods, is healthiest in the long term, so don't avoid reintroducing ordinary foods unless there's good reason. Do try to steer clear of highly processed and 'junk' foods now your body has become used to living without them, and go easy on alcohol and caffeine.

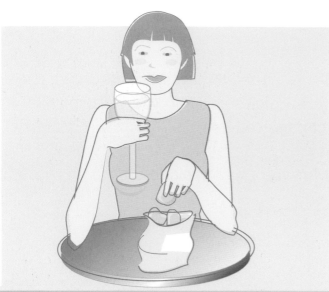

1 are you:
a) Overweight?
b) About the right weight?
c) Underweight?

2 do you eat highly processed foods, white carbs, 'junk' foods:
a) Every day?
b) Fairly frequently?
c) Rarely or never?

do you need a detox?

If you're still wavering about whether you should try a detox or not, answer these ten questions and then check your score ....

how long should a detox last?
Some people do a 2- or 3-day detox once a month, others do a week every 3 months, others a month once or twice a year. My own experience shows that a 'grade 1' detox should only be carried out for up to a week, while a more moderate detox can be beneficial for a month or so.

Doing a detox for just a day or two is really a short-term crash diet by any other name, and while it may help you to feel less guilty about pigging out last weekend, is unlikely to achieve a great deal in the way of ridding your body of pollutants. Pollutants such as heavy metals and drug residues are stored in body fat, which cannot be got rid of in a few days, as we are all painfully aware!

3 do you drink alcohol:
a) Every day?
b) Several times a week?
c) Rarely or never?

4 thinking about your lifestyle, your job, your overall stress levels, are you:
a) Living a very stressful life?
b) Stressed sometimes but not all the time?
c) Rarely stressed?

5 on most days, do you feel:
a) Tired all the time and very lethargic?
b) Usually OK, but get tired easily?
c) Full of energy and enthusiasm?

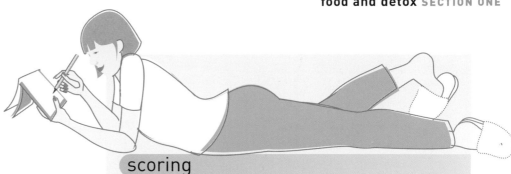

6 how strongly do you feel that you need to change and/or refresh your life?

a) Very strongly?
b) Moderately so?
c) Not at all?

7 compared with other areas of your life, how much attention have you paid recently to your diet:

a) Hardly any?
b) A fair amount of attention?
c) A great deal?

8 How would you rate the condition of your skin (appearance, texture):

a) Very poor?
b) Average?
c) Very good?

9 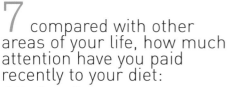 do you have gum problems, such as bleeding or inflammation:

a) All the time?
b) Now and then?
c) Rarely or never?

10 looking at your eyes in a mirror in daylight are they:

a) Tired, bloodshot or yellow-tinged?
b) Not too bad for your age?
c) White whites, sparkling and alert?

scoring

Give yourself 3 points for every A, 2 points for every B, and 1 point for every C. Add up your total.

If you scored 25–30:
You are in dire need of a mind and body detox. You need to recognize that you and your body are as important as, if not more important than, any other factors in your life. You may feel you haven't time to put yourself on a detox programme, but you need it more than most. Make the time – start the detox programme overleaf, either for a long weekend or take a week's holiday and do it then. While doing it, try to be self-aware and learn ways to treat yourself as you deserve to be treated. Couple your diet detox with a gentle exercise programme (see Section 2) and plenty of relaxation. Try to build the things the detox teaches you into your everyday life on a permanent basis.

If you scored 11–24:
You probably eat reasonably well and feel that you have your life under control – but take care; in mid life it is harder to maintain optimum levels of energy and health unless you spend real time understanding the changing needs of your body. You could benefit from a gentle detox –– try the programme overleaf (moderate version) for a week and note the differences in how you feel. A week like this once a month would probably produce more benefits and help you change your food choices for the better every day of the year.

If you scored 10 or under:
You could be an extremely healthy and perfect example of how to manage yourself and your life as you head into middle age – in which case, very well done. Few people live an exemplary life, even if they know what they should be doing! It is unlikely that you need a detox diet – in fact, if you are underweight, a serious detox is not for you, as the calorie content is almost always low.

A word of warning: if anyone has ever described you as a 'health fanatic' or perhaps a 'health food freak', or if you agree with either description of yourself, take care – there is evidence that it can be as unhealthy to be obsessive or borderline obsessive about your health regime as it is to be a couch-potato junk-food junkie!

the detox diet

The 7-day Grade 1 detox plan here can also be used for just 3 or 4 days if you prefer (pick the first 3 or last 4 days). The moderate detox at the bottom of the opposite page can be done for 1 week up to six times a year, 2 weeks up to four times a year or for a month up to twice a year. Alternatively, devise your own plan using the list of 'dos' and don'ts' opposite.

instructions

● Follow the Grade 1 diet for up to 1 week only and for no more than six times a year.

● Drink 8 glasses of water daily (or replace some of the water with green or white tea). Space these out evenly throughout the day. On rising every day, have a drink of hot water with the juice of half a lemon and 2 teaspoons runny honey.

● Have 2 between-meal snacks daily, one of 5–10 fresh almonds, Brazil nuts or walnuts, the other of I tablespoon of pumpkin or sun-flower seeds.

● All salad leaves are unlimited.

● Try to ensure that all the food you eat is organic.

● Have portions according to your appetite, size and exercise levels.

● Avoid long periods of vigorous exercise while on the Grade 1 detox (it doesn't provide enough calories) – stick to moderate periods of aero-bic exercise like walking, breast-stroke swimming or moderate-paced cycling, and other forms of exercise such as yoga or stretching.

● Support the detox with regular baths or showers, body-brushing and at least an hour a day of 'self' – meditation, massage and so on.

day 1

breakfast
Fresh fruit salad (no added sugar, use fresh fruit juice or water to moisten)

lunch
Salad of mixed dark-green and red leaves with a handful of fresh herbs of choice (chopped or torn) dressed with olive oil French dressing,
$1/2$ avocado sliced in
Slice of watermelon

evening
1 medium bowl of home-made lentil soup (using brown, green or Puy lentils, salt-free veg stock and chopped onion – simmer for 45 minutes then purée if you prefer and reheat)
1 apple

day 2

breakfast
Fruit smoothie made by blending a selection of soft fruits (e.g. berries, bananas, mango, peach or nectarine) with some water to make a thick drink (add a little runny honey if you like)

lunch
2 tablespoons home-made or best-quality hummus
2 salt-free brown rice cakes
Large salad of leaves as Day One (exclude the avocado) sprinkled with 1 dessertspoon pine nuts

evening
1 medium bowl of home-made vegetable soup using any orange or red veg (chop, simmer in salt-free vegetable stock for 45 minutes then purée if you prefer and reheat)

day 3

breakfast
2 tablespoons wheat-free oat-based muesli with 1 chopped apple and soya milk
1 slice of watermelon

lunch
1 bowl of vegetable soup as Day 2
2 unsalted brown rice cakes

evening
Large sliced tomato, red onion and basil salad with 1 tablespoon olive oil French dressing beaten with 1 table-spoon good-quality guacamole and sprinkled with 1 dessertspoon linseeds

day 4

As Day 1

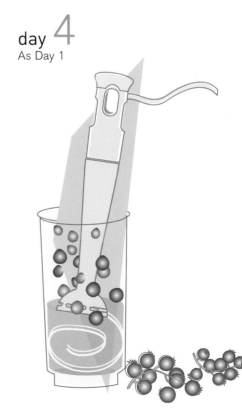

day 5

breakfast
1 apple and 1 orange, each segmented and arranged with 1 small sliced banana, all drizzled with 2 teaspoons runny honey

lunch
1 bowl of lentil soup as Day 1
1 medium slice of dark rye bread

evening
Salad of cucumber, peppers, tomato, red onion, fresh coriander leaves and black olives dressed with 1 tablespoon olive oil mixed with 1 dessertspoon balsamic vinegar and black pepper
5 Brazil nuts

day 6

breakfast
As Day 2

lunch
Purée of cooked butter beans with lemon juice, olive oil and black pepper, with 2 unsalted brown rice cakes
Large mixed salad of choice with olive oil French dressing
1 apple

evening
Selection of Mediterranean veg (e.g courgettes, aubergines, red onions, beef tomatoes), sliced, drizzled with olive oil and black pepper, and roasted for 45 minutes with a few whole garlic cloves (drizzle over more oil and lemon juice mixed with a little light tahini to serve)
1 slice of dark rye bread

day 7

As Day 3

DIY grade 1 detox

Follow this list of foods to use and foods to avoid to devise your own detox. The section at the bottom shows add-ons for longer-term use (see the introduction)

foods to go for
All fruits (including a few dried fruits, if you like, but make sure they are organic), preferably raw but occasionally lightly cooked is fine. Fresh fruit smoothies are preferable to extracted juices as they retain more nutrients, but juice is fine now and then.

● All vegetables, raw or lightly cooked (e.g. steamed or stir-fried in olive oil), or used in a soup or casserole. All salad items, raw.

● All pulses (e.g. lentils, chickpeas, cannellini beans, black-eye beans), dried and cooked, or use good-quality canned in water; sprouted pulses, soya milk.

● All fresh herbs (e.g. parsley, rosemary, thyme, sage, chervil, basil, coriander, dill). All fresh spices (e.g. ginger) and dried whole spices (e.g. black pepper).

● Good-quality pure olive oil, groundnut oil, walnut oil, sesame oil.

● Fresh nuts and seeds, organic peanut butter, tahini.

● Brown basmati rice, brown unsalted rice cakes, dark rye bread, rolled oats.

● Top-quality pure, single-source organic runny honey, preferably manuka.

● Salt-free, artificial-additive-free vegetable stock.

foods to avoid

● Meat, poultry, fish, dairy produce, eggs.

● Sugar and all processed carbohydrate foods, including white bread, white rice.

● Highly processed foods containing additives; long-life heat-treated foods.

● Wheat and wheat-based products, including wheat bread, wheat breakfast cereals, cakes, biscuits, pastry, wheat pasta.

● Foods with added salt. (If doing a lot of exercise in hot weather you may need a mineral-balanced energy drink to supply essential body salts.)

● Alcohol and caffeine-rich drinks, such as coffee, strong tea, cola; all fizzy drinks and diet drinks.

▶ **Moderate detox** Add these foods into your menus on the Grade 1 detox for a more gentle regime, higher in calories and protein (all foods should be organic): ● Chicken and game ● White fish, oily fish ● Low-fat bio yoghurt ● Also, have up to 2 slices of dark rye bread a day in addition to those listed in the 7-day diet.

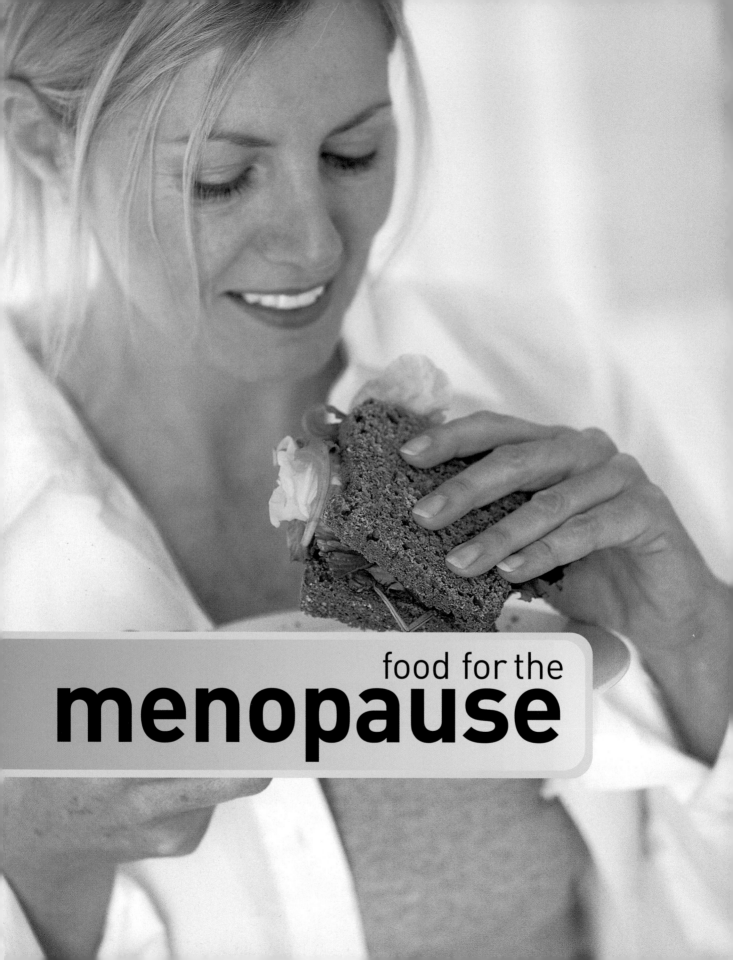

food for the
menopause

There is much that women can do through diet to combat the side-effects and possible negative health effects of the menopause. As worries over taking HRT seem to escalate, with two out of three women giving HRT drugs up within a year of starting them, dietary intervention may be the sensible way to go. On these pages we look at the many links between diet and menopausal health, as well as examining the truth behind the headlines, and finally there is a blueprint menopausal diet.

The time around and after the female menopause is linked with several health problems, some potentially serious. The feature on Menopause and Andropause in Section 4 – Well-being for Your New Life – discusses the menopause in more general terms. Here we look at whether or not your diet can minimize the risks and influence the outcome.

weight gain
As we saw earlier in this section, too much weight gain in mid life is associated with an increased risk of health problems. Very many women report that they gain most weight during and immediately after the menopause. Until recently, most studies on the subject came to the conclusion that the menopause itself wasn't responsible for this increase and that it was simply that women at this time exercised less, or that it was a continuation of the gradual decline in metabolic rate that happens to us all after about 35.

Two more recent studies indicate that women ARE right when they say that the menopause piles on extra pounds even if they eat no more and exercise just as much.

One found that menopausal women put on about 2 pounds extra a year without any changes in diet or lifestyle, due to a sudden decrease in metabolic rate, while a study published in the *Journal of Clinical Endocrinology* found that changes in the way body fat is metabolized predisposes post-menopausal women to gain fat around the stomach and bottom.

In view of these findings it seems even more important to eat a healthy diet, moderate in calories and fat, in order to try to limit the amount of weight that is gained. Advice on the menopause and exercise is on page 177.

bone loss
The demineralization of your bones speeds up at menopause by 600%, due largely to the huge decrease in the hormone oestrogen circulating in the body, and this may result in osteoporosis later in life. Indeed, one in five people over the age of 60 have the disease.

Much can be done to protect the bones via diet (see Around 50, page 16). There has been a great deal written in the past few years about using plant oestrogens to maintain bone density in the menopause. These phyto-oestrogens have a mildly oestrogenic effect within the body which, some experts think, will replace natural oestrogen at the menopause and after.

However, the UK Government's Committee on Toxicology (COT) reported in 2003 that, although short-term studies of high plant oestrogen diets suggest a small protective effect in the spine, there is little scientific evidence in humans for their usefulness. Trials using rodents, on the other hand, have consistently shown that diets high in soya or other isoflavones (a group of phyto-oestrogens) DO help prevent bone loss.

The COT concludes that more human trials need to be done, while the UK Food Standards Agency (FSA) advises that the amount of plant oestrogens needed in the diet in order to have even a small effect on the bones would be so great that it isn't an effective treatment for osteoporosis. That said, a 2002 scientific study reported in the *Journal of Bone and Mineral Research* found that supplementation with 54mg a day of genistein (a type of isoflavone) was as successful as HRT in maintaining bone health.

It may soon be proved that supplements are the answer. In the meantime, a diet rich in phyto-oestrogens MAY help your bones and could be worth trying, especially if osteoporosis runs in your family. However, if you have – or are at risk from – breast or other hormonal cancers, the FSA advises that you DON'T eat a high-oestrogenic diet or take supplements.

cardiovascular (CV) disease

Once women have been through the menopause, their risk of contracting any of the diseases of the cardiovascular system increases to the same level as that of men. This is because they no longer have the protection that the female hormones appear to offer. A diet rich in antioxidants (see page 19), omega-3 fats, fruit, vegetables, whole grains and pulses, and maintaining a reasonable weight, can offer protection against CV diseases. Regular intake of soya beans or products has been shown to offer protection from heart disease and, in the US, manufacturers are allowed to make such health claims on labelling. Supplementation with isoflavones extracted from soya beans doesn't show similar levels of protection.

For other menopausal symptoms, see individual articles;
▶ Dry skin, page 126;
▶ Hair condition, page 146–8;
▶ Lack of libido, page 179;
▶ Poor memory, page 203
▶ Tiredness and insomnia, page 186–9;
▶ Mood swings and anxiety, see Mind Matters, page 199;
▶ Joint aches and pains and headaches, pages 190–91.

cancers: After menopause, there is increased risk of breast cancer. Overweight is a major risk factor for breast cancer, and high alcohol intake also increases risk. Some research appears to show high intake of plant oestrogens can reduce risk, while others show increased risk. The UK's COT report on phyto-oestrogens concluded there is some evidence for their beneficial effects on both breast and prostate cancer based upon animal experiments, while the Food Standards Agency's advice is that people at high risk of breast or prostate cancer should NOT eat a diet high in phyto-oestrogens. Confusing or what?

More research on humans has to be done and, meanwhile, it is probably wise to eat an overall balanced, healthy diet (e.g. the Menopause Eating Plan overleaf) with moderate intakes of the oestro-genic plant foods unless you have been specifically advised otherwise. If you think you may be at high risk of breast cancer (if one or more of your family has had it), you should talk to your doctor.

menopausal symptoms

Hot flushes Probably the worst symptom for many, no one knows exactly what causes them, but they can be minimized or made worse by diet.
AVOID Drinking very hot drinks, alcohol, high-caffeine drinks, hot and spicy meals.
GO FOR A diet high in fresh fruits, veg, salads, whole grains and pulses. This will provide an increase in plant oestrogens, which appear to minimize flushes in some women. Regular cool water or teas; vitamin B group and E supplements. Some women report reduction in flushes using red clover, agnus castus and/or sage supplements; others swear by evening primrose oil. Black cohosh is no longer advised by many experts as it can have unwanted side-effects.

What are phyto-oestrogens? They are compounds found in many plants which have an oestrogen-like effect in the body. They can be divided into flavonoids and non-flavonoids. The flavonoids are subdivided into isoflavones, such as genistein and daidzein (found mainly in pulses such as soya beans, chickpeas and lentils) and coumestans, such as coumestrol (found mainly in sprouted pulses). The non-flavonoids are lignans, found in seeds, whole grains and fresh fruits and vegetables.

top 10 menopause managers

1. **brazil nuts** High in selenium, which can improve the condition of dry skin and hair, increase the action of the thyroid gland and help protect against heart disease. Other nuts are also useful sources.

2. **fish** Oily fish, such as salmon and mackerel, is high in omega-3 fatty acids to help minimize joint pain, risk of heart disease and some cancers, and improve skin and hair condition. Shellfish is high in zinc, may help to increase libido and is a powerful antioxidant.

3. **low-fat dairy produce** Contains calcium for healthy bones, heart and nerves, which is better absorbed when high amounts of saturated fat aren't present but small amounts of omega-3 or -6 fats are present.

4. **flax seeds (linseeds)** High in phyto-oestrogens called lignans, these may reduce hot flushes, may block cancer cells in certain conditions and are one of the few non fish sources of omega-3s, which have a host of benefits.

5. **whole grains** Whole grains, such as barley, rye and oats, contain lignans (see Flax seeds above) and other types of phytochemicals that can help protect you from heart disease and cancers.

6. **spices** ginger is the most useful spice for helping to alleviate headaches and bloating; turmeric is another spice which can help minimize painful joint and other aches and pains of the menopause.

7. **herbal remedies** St John's Wort can ease depression, a common side-effect of the menopause, while gingko biloba may help your memory and agnus castus can help relieve hot flushes.

8. **supplements** Evening primrose oil is rich in the longer-chain omega-6 fatty acids and some women report good results (which are not quick to kick in, nevertheless) using a daily supplement for menopausal symptoms. Vitamins B6 and calcium supplements have been shown to improve mood and sleep in some women.

9. **tofu, soya and other pulses** Rich in plant oestrogens called isoflavones (of which there are many subdivisions, including genistein and daidzein) which can help to prevent heart disease, lower blood cholesterol, may possibly help to prevent breast cancer and are said to help alleviate hot flushes and other menopausal symptoms. If you like baking, use soya flour or at least partially replace wheat flour.

10. **beansprouts** Alfalfa and mung beansprouts are rich in coumestans, another type of natural plant oestrogen. Chinese herbalists use alfalfa sprouts for menopausal symptoms.

menopause eating plan

The 7-day eating plan shown here should help to reduce the symptoms of the menopause, such as hot flushes, sweats, tiredness and aches and pains. The diet contains a moderately high amount of natural plant oestrogens and, if you are at risk of breast cancer or actually have breast cancer, you should seek advice from your doctor before embarking on the plan.

instructions

● Follow the plan as laid out, having portion sizes to suit your appetite, unless you are overweight, in which case try to have moderate portions only.

● Eat your between-meal snacks, as eating little and often may produce fewer hot flushes than eating one big meal less frequently.

● Have about 8 glasses of water a day, or iced white, green or weak black tea can be used to replace 3–4 of these glasses.

● Take any herbal or vitamin supplements you are trying with water, along with a meal or snack.

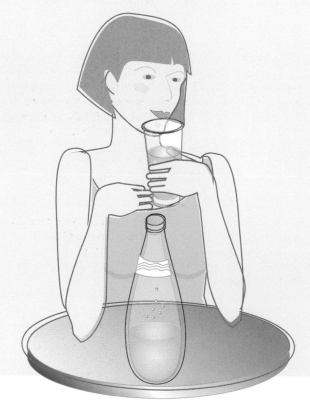

breakfast every day

should be one of the following options:
1 A bowlful of good-quality muesli with oat flakes, rye flakes, nuts, seeds and dried fruits, with a selection of fresh fruit of your choice chopped or sprinkled in, with 1 level dessertspoon flax seeds, and covered with calcium-enriched soya milk.
2 A bowl of calcium-enriched soya yoghurt, 3–4 tablespoons fruit compote (e.g. apple, plum, or mixed reconstituted dried fruit), sprinkled with muesli as above and topped with flax seeds.
NOTE: Skimmed milk and low-fat bio yoghurt can be substituted for the soya milk if you prefer, or do this every other day.

snacks

Every day have TWO between-meal snacks consisting of one of the following – try to vary your choices as much as possible:
● 5 Brazil nuts or 8 almonds
● I level dessertspoon sunflower seeds or pumpkin seeds
● 1 tablespoon good-quality hummus on 1 dark rye crispbread
● 1 dessertspoon tahini on 1 organic brown rice cake
● 4 pieces of organic dried apricot or 2 dried figs
● 1 small pot fruit calcium-enriched fruit soya yoghurt

day 1

lunch

Brown basmati rice and chickpea salad with your choice of chopped salad vegetables and fresh herbs added, and dressed in olive oil French dressing
Pot of low-fat bio fromage frais or soya yoghurt with runny honey and 1 teaspoon sunflower seeds

evening

Grilled herring fillets
Orange and chicory salad
Broccoli
Rye bread with low-fat spread

day 2

lunch

Sandwich of 2 slices of dark rye bread filled with ripe avocado and slices of half-fat mozzarella cheese, plus salad items
Apple or peach

evening

Casserole of pot barley, mixed root vegetables and tofu
Stir-fried spring greens
10 almonds

day 3

lunch

Tomato and basil soup
Soft goats' cheese
3 oatcakes
1 orange or kiwi fruit

evening

Casserole of pot barley, mixed root vegetables and tofu
Stir-fried spring greens
10 almonds

day 4

lunch

Wholemeal pitta bread filled with hummus and mixed salad
Piece of fruit of choice

evening

Grilled or poached salmon steak
1 dessertspoon home-made green pesto
Green lentils
Stir-fried red peppers in olive oil

day 5

lunch

Feta cheese
Dark rye crispbreads
Side salad of walnuts, celery and apple dressed with olive oil French dressing

evening

1 pack of mixed frozen seafood, defrosted and stir-fried in olive oil before tossing with 2–3 tablespoons of good-quality tomato and basil pasta sauce before reheating. Serve on brown basmati rice
Broccoli
1 piece of fruit of choice

day 6

lunch

Sandwich of 2 slices of dark rye bread filled with organic sugar-free peanut butter, rocket and other salad leaves of choice
Cherry tomato and spring onion salad
5 Brazil nuts

evening

Small lean beef steak, grilled
New potatoes
Green beans
Spinach

day 7

lunch

Salad of fresh beansprouts, grated carrot, green beans and sweetcorn, dressed in olive oil French dressing into which you have beaten a little silken tofu
1 slice of dark rye bread
5 almonds

evening

Chicken, tomato and thyme casserole
Brown basmati rice or quinoa
Steamed greens or spinach
Peas

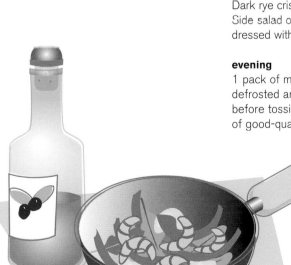

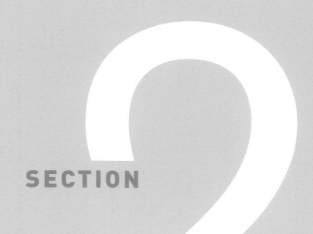

SECTION **2**

body for your
newlife

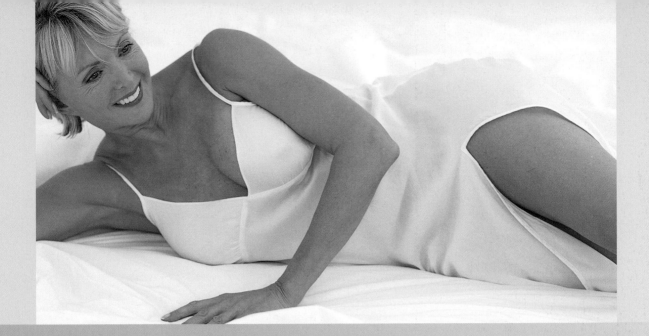

If you want to feel good – if you want to grab life by the tails – you need your body to be in good working order. The most simple key to achieving this is to take regular exercise, and yet 75% of people aged 50 and over don't take any real exercise at all.

There is a wealth of scientific research to show that keeping active and keeping fit are among the very best ways to stay in good health as we get older. In Section 2, we will be examining all the links between exercise, feeling good and health protection, and showing you how best to use exercise to enhance your life.

Around the age of 50 and 60, many people feel it's too late to begin getting more active, but that is not true. Your body is amazingly adept at coping with new demands on it – as long as you are sensible – and studies show that older bodies make improvements in fitness and appearance just as rapidly as younger ones.

If food is your body's fuel, then exercise is the catalyst that keeps you running smoothly, efficiently and without problems … for the rest of your life.

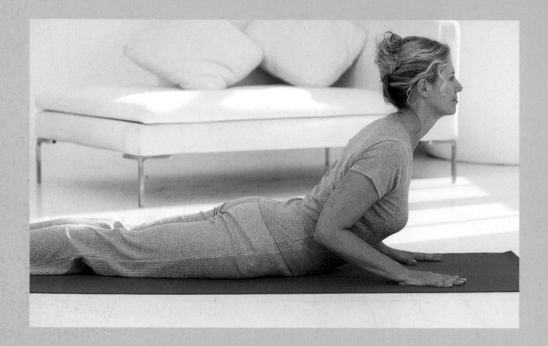

use it or lose it! That could be the mantra for your body's health. We look at all the ways in which exercise can help you feel great.

If you're in any doubt that you could benefit from regular activity, try the body questionnaire on the following pages. You need only carry out a few simple exercises, taking a few minutes of your time, then add up your score to find out how old your body really is. Most of us over 40 will probably be shocked to find that whatever the calendar says, our real age is older. The older you are in 'real' terms, the more your body is crying out for exercise.

For a healthy heart, take regular exercise. So much research has now been done to prove this link beyond doubt. Indeed, an eight-year study of 22,000 men in the USA found fitness was of greater importance in maintaining heart health than being slim, so if you are fat but fit you'll live longer than if you're slim but unfit. Most studies show daily walking can reduce risk of heart disease by up to 50%. Similar results have been shown in beating strokes and high blood pressure, and in improving blood fat and cholesterol profiles.

Studies also link inactivity with increased risk of Type-2 diabetes and some cancers – for example, exercise cuts the risk of bowel cancer by a third.

Among the most obvious signs of ageing are a thickening waist, a pot belly, poor posture and lumps and bumps where before there were none. However, regular exercise can reverse most of these signs – if not helping you revert to exactly how you used to be, then at least making huge improvements. Improving your shape can also improve your health – for example, reducing your pot belly or 'apple' shape can reduce your risk of heart disease.

People who take regular exercise also find it much easier to stay slim than those who don't. This is even more important if you have dieted to lose weight. A US study of slimmers five years on from dieting found that the 70% who had kept all or most of their weight off had taken part in regular activities throughout that time. All the available evidence says that the weight will return unless you are active.

If you feel tired you take a rest, but there is a lot of evidence to show that the best way to feel better and more energized is to do the reverse ... go out for a walk, or take other light aerobic exercise such as swimming. Exercise increases the blood flow to the brain and releases hormones that help you to feel better, as well as increasing brain power and lifting depression.

If you have a moderate backache or arthritis, tense shoulders or unspecified aches and pains – again, rather than rest, research shows that you should exercise. This will loosen up ligaments and joints, strengthen the muscles that support the bone structure and benefit your body in several other ways.

Moreover, regular weight-bearing activity can increase bone density and minimize the risk of osteoporosis and fractures.

Even if you have trouble relaxing or getting to sleep, if you suffer from insomnia or stress, all forms of exercise will help you to relax. Activity literally releases the tension in your body, as well as sending calming hormones where they need to be.

In the pages that follow you'll find what type of exercise to do to beat your own particular problems. I hope to prove exercising can be fun – and safe, whatever your age or fitness level.

how old is your body?

Your age in years may be 40, 50 or 60 – but how old is your body? Take the tests on these pages and find out whether you're really a toned 20-year-old or a sagging 70. However young at heart you are, without a reasonably fit body you aren't going to feel as young as you could. The 10 tests here are easily and quickly done and the results will give you a good estimate of your true physical age.

what to do   To carry out the tests wear suitable, comfortable clothing, such as a lightweight tracksuit or T-shirt and shorts, and wear trainers. Try to do the tests in a warm room when you are feeling well, not too soon after a meal.

You will need a watch with a second hand or timer, pen and paper, a tape measure, a stair or step, a flat wall that you can stand against, a ruler and someone to help for the last test. It would be helpful if you have someone with you throughout the tests, to assess how you do, though this isn't essential.

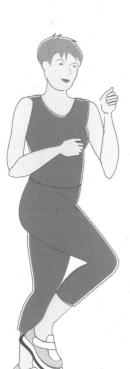

1 stamina test – step-ups

● Stand in front of a portable step or a stair 6–8 inches (15–20cm) high. Step up with the left foot, then bring up the right. Take the left foot back down, then the right. That counts as one step.
● Step up and down like this for 1 minute and count how many you do.

0 – 15 Add 10 years to your age
16 – 25 Add 5 years
26 – 35 Add nothing
36 – 50 Subtract 2 years
51+ Subtract 5 years

2 upper-body strength test – press-ups

● Upper-body strength and tone often get ignored. Lie on your front, placing both hands at shoulder level but outside each one. Keeping the toes on floor and elbows below shoulder height, push into your palms to raise the upper body so that your back is flat. Return your body to the floor and repeat.
● How many can you do in one minute?

0 – 15 Add 2 years
16 – 25 Add nothing
26+ Subtract 5 years

3 lower-body strength test – squats

● Stand with feet hip-width apart, arms out in front of you, then bend knees and lower bottom as if you were going to sit down, until your thighs are parallel to the floor. Return to starting position.
● Count how many you can do in 1 minute.

0 – 15 Add 5 years
16 – 30 Add 2 years
31 – 40 Add nothing
40+ Subtract 2 years

4 abdominal strength test – sit-ups

● Lie on your back on a mat with feet on the floor, knees bent and arms at your sides. Breathing out, slowly lift head and neck (and back if possible) off the floor and allow your arms to slide forward.
● Record how far your arms reach. Return to floor. SAFETY NOTE: Only go as far as you are able without undue strain. If you have a bad back, don't perform this exercise but add 5 years to your count.

Can't perform – Add 10 years
Wrists go to thighs – Add 5 years
Elbows go to thighs – Add nothing
Chest reaches thighs – Subtract 5 years

5 flexibility test 1 – sit-and-reach

● Bodily stiffness, lack of flexibility in the joints and a narrow range of movement are all associated with ageing. This measures flexibility in the lower back and hamstrings, two of the first areas to stiffen with age.
● Sit on a mat with your legs straight out in front of you, hip-width apart and feet flexed, arms at your sides and lower back not slumped. Stretch out your arms towards your toes. How far can you go and HOLD for a minimum count of three? NOTE: DO NOT round out the lower back to try to reach further.

No further than mid-to-lower leg – Add 5 years
Around ankles – Add 2 years
To the toes but no further – Add nothing
Beyond the toes – Subtract 3 years

6 flexibility test 2 – sit-and-twist

● Spinal flexibility is important for enabling you to do so many of the typical activities of youth, like dancing and some more exotic sexual positions. Sit on a mat on the floor with back straight and legs out in front of you, feet flexed. Place right hand, palm flat, on the floor behind your lower spine and then twist shoulders around so that you're looking over your right shoulder. Hold for 10 seconds.

Couldn't twist shoulders at all – Add 5 years
Could twist a little but not enough to look over shoulder – Add 2 years
Could twist as described – Subtract 5 years

7 weight test

● Most people gain weight as they get older. How much weight have you put on since you were 25?

More than 3 stones – Add 5 years
1–3 stones – Add 2 years
Less than a stone – Add nothing

8 waist circumference test

● Your waist measurement is an excellent indication of your physical condition.

Your waist measures over 40 inches (1 metre) if male or over 34 1/2 inches (87cm) if female? – Add 3 years
Your waist measures over 37 inches (93cm) if male or over 31 1/2 inches (79cm) if female? – Add 1 year
All other measurements – Add nothing

9 posture test

Poor posture is a classic giveaway of age and can add years to the slimmest of bodies.
● Stand with your back against a wall. Can you stand with the back of your head, your shoulders, your tailbone and your heels all touching the wall at the same time?

No – Add 3 years.
Yes – Subtract 3 years

10 reflex test

Slowing reflexes are one of the main reasons that older people have to give up competitive sports, but you can keep them sharp with regular practice. Try this test.
● Stand facing a helper with your hands extended and 6 inches (15cm) apart. Get your helper to hold a ruler between your hands, with the 1 inch (1cm) mark at the bottom and level with your hands, and the 12 inch (30cm) mark at the top.
● Now your helper should drop the ruler and you should try to catch it immediately. Repeat 6 times.
● How many times did you manage to catch the ruler before the 2 inch (5cm) mark?

Not at all – Add 3 years
1–2 times – Add 2 years
3 times – Add nothing
4 times – Subtract 1 year
5 times – Subtract 2 years

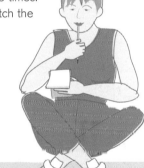

working out your score

Total up all the additions and write the number here: _____

Total up all the subtractions and write the number here: _____

Take away the smallest number from the greatest and add this final total to your current age (or subtract it if your subtractions total is the larger number) to give you your true body age.
For example: you are currently aged 50, your total of additions is 20 and your total of subtractions is 12. You have 8 more additions than subtractions, so your true body age is 58.
As you work through this section in the months ahead, your true body age should improve.

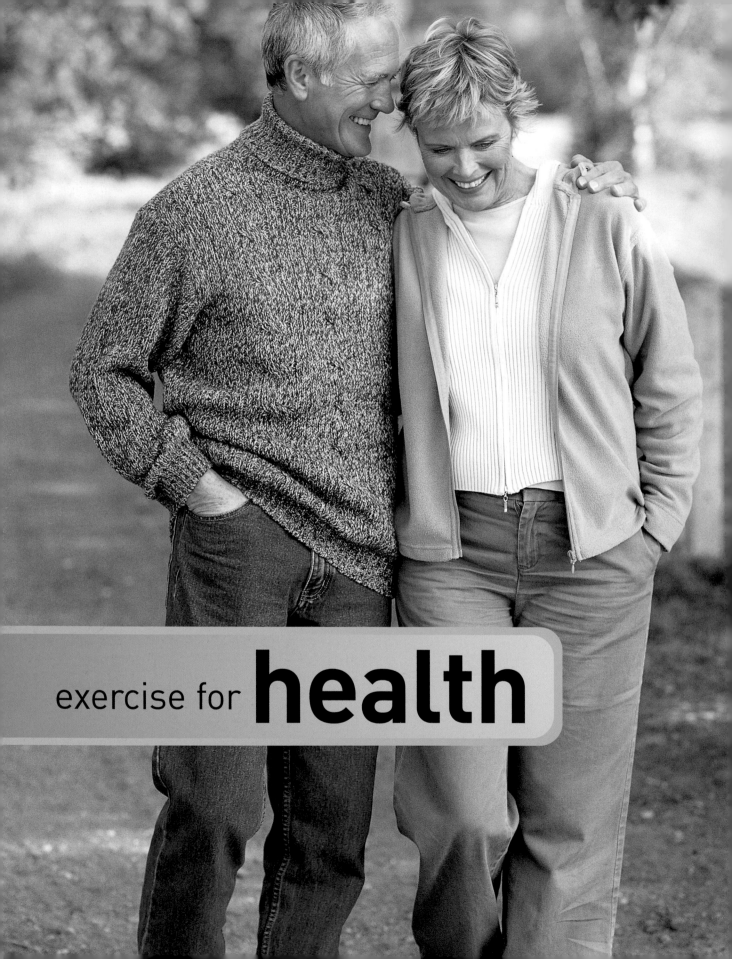

exercise for **health**

'Enough evidence exists relating sedentary habits to poor health to classify physical inactivity as a major risk factor for early death.' So say the authors of one of the most authoritative books ever on exercise, *Essentials of Exercise Physiology*. They also say that regular exercise throughout your life provides significant protection from coronary heart disease and stroke, and that people who do even mild exercise report better health than sedentary people.

Cardiovascular diseases cause approximately half of all deaths in mid-lifers and the elderly in the USA and UK, and yet regular moderate exercise can reduce the risks by up to 50%, by reducing the heart rate, helping to reduce high blood pressure and improving the profile of blood fats.

Exercise, it is clear, also enhances health in other ways. A cardiovascular system made fit through regular activity can also help protect us against cancer, type-2 diabetes and obesity, while a study of 17,000 Harvard University students showed that regular exercise counters the effects of cigarette smoking and excess body weight.

regular exercise
Interestingly, for unfit people it takes only small improvements in the amount of exercise they do to reap important benefits. The regularity, rather than the intensity, is what counts most. Several studies show that 20–30 minutes of walking four times a week can be enough to make a great difference in your health profile.

● A study published in the *Journal of the American Medical Association* found that women who walked for half an hour a day had a 30% less chance of stroke.

● A study published in the *New England Journal of Medicine* found that walking is as good as running in reducing the risk of cardiovascular disease (CVD) for women aged 50–79.

● And in adults with diabetes, regular walking of two hours a week lowered the death rates from all causes by 39%.

never too late
Whether you are 40 or 60 – or even 80 – research shows that you can improve your fitness levels and health considerably after only a few weeks or months of exercise. One study from Texas, which monitored a group of men at age 20 and then 30 years later, found that by the age of 50 the men had become unfit and flabby – but that after a programme of regular aerobic exercise their fitness profiles had returned to the same levels they had had at 20.

The consensus of professional opinion is that in mid life a healthy adult can get the aerobic capacity of a fit person 20–25 years younger with regular effort, however unfit at the outset.

what to do
In order to improve your health and chances of living a long life, you simply need to do regular aerobic exercise – this is exercise which increases your heart rate. The programmes overleaf will all achieve this in a total of 1–2 hours a week. For people of poor or moderate fitness, 90 minutes a week is plenty. Add to that a few of our suggested lifestyle changes and within three months you should see significant improvement.

the plans
On the following pages we have three simple staged programmes to increase your cardiovascular fitness for the benefits we talked about on the previous page. Before beginning any of them, read the tips in the introduction below.

make your workout work for you

If you exercise too hard – especially if you haven't exercised much or at all in the recent past – it could be dangerous, but if on the other hand you don't push yourself hard enough, you won't improve your fitness level and gain the associated health benefits.

So it's best to aim for a quite steady state of 'moderate-to-hard' exertion during your workout. This means that you can just about talk comfortably while you are working out. If you can't talk, you are working too hard; if you find you can chat easily, however, you are obviously not working hard enough.

For a slightly more scientific test, you can if you like purchase a heart rate monitor (these are widely available from sports shops or via the Internet) and use this to make sure that your heart rate is between 50% and 70% of your maximum during your workout. Maximum heart rate (MHR) equals 220 minus your age for women, or 226 minus your age for men. For example, if you are female and aged 50 your MHR is 170; 50% of that is 85, 60% is 102, while 70% is 119.

In the early stages of an aerobic fitness programme for older adults who haven't exercised in a while, it is best to start at the 50% level (i.e. keeping your heart rate at around this level throughout your workout) and then to increase this up through 60% and 70% as the weeks progress.

Before you start, and at all stages throughout, do bear in mind the safety suggestions that are listed opposite.

See also:
▶ For all cool-down stretches, see the panel on pages 82–3.

▶ **Did you know ...?**

● You can buy rubbery knobbled insoles for sports shoes that absorb much more shock than standard trainers and are ideal for people prone to knee or ankle injury and joint pain.

● You don't need an array of special supplements to help you work better when training. There is some scientific evidence to show, though, that co-enzyme Q10 may help unfit people work for longer.

● The US College of Sports Medicine recommends up to 600ml of water 2 hours before exercising and an extra 150ml for each 20 minutes of aerobic exercise.

● Some research shows that if you feel very tired during or after a work-out, it may not just be because you are unfit. You could be short of iron in your diet – so eat more red meat, whole grains and dark leafy greens, eggs and dried fruit.

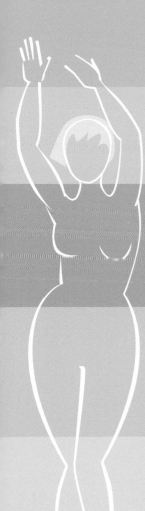

safety at any age

● Check with your doctor before beginning an exercise programme.

● For people who are unfit or have any health problems, it is usually best to start with the walking programme, but your own physician will help you decide.

● People with problems like arthritis or chronic back pain should follow an aerobic exercise programme personally recommended to them by a doctor or exercise professional. This programme may be suitable – show it to them and see.

● The Questionnaire on pages 64–5 will help you determine your fitness level.

● For each programme, start at Level 1 and work up gradually through the levels at your own pace.

● Warm up before and cool down after each aerobic exercise session. If you don't, you may risk muscular pain and possible faintness or dizziness afterwards.

● Wear good training shoes which absorb shock. Wear comfortable clothes that allow unrestricted movement for walking and cycling – tracksuit bottoms and a T-shirt are ideal.

● Monitor your exertion level while exercising (see opposite).

● Have a small snack about an hour before exercising, and don't forget to take a small water bottle with you.

● Be sensible! Start on a level that is right for you.

everyday exercise

To maximize the benefits of your structured programme, try to think of ways of increasing your activity levels in your everyday life. Research shows that you can almost double the amount of exercise you take by adopting even a few of these ideas:

● Whenever you are walking (e.g. round the shops, to the newsagent), make an effort to speed up to a 'training' level.

● When using the car, park a little further away from where you want to be – most people try to park as close as possible.

● Use stairs whenever you can, and avoid lifts and escalators.

● Add ankle weights for walking around.

● When you have waiting time (e.g. while cooking), use it to do some on-the-spot moves (e.g. marching on the spot).

● If you have music on at home, don't just sit or stand and listen – dance to it.

● If watching TV in the evening, don't sit there for hours but get up and move around every 15 minutes or so. Use the ads to do a small chore (e.g. finish the washing up). If you build activity into your regular life it becomes second nature.

walking programme

Warm up by walking slowly or marching on spot for 3 minutes. ● Work through the levels in your own time. If you prefer, you can have Day 7 off each week, just doing three walks a week, but your progress will be slower.

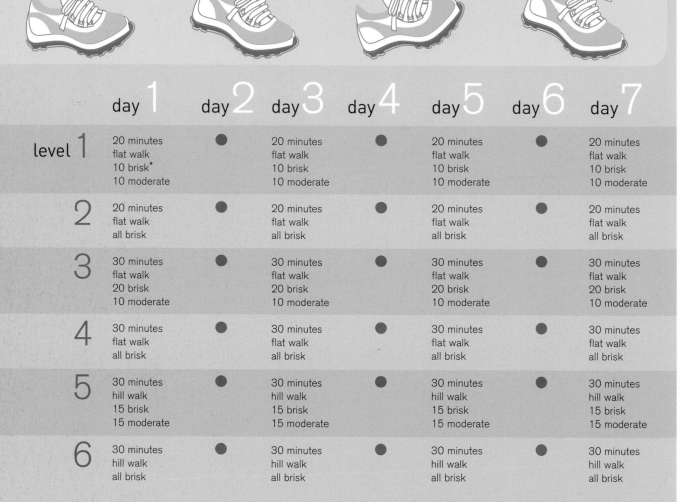

	day 1	day 2	day 3	day 4	day 5	day 6	day 7
level 1	20 minutes flat walk 10 brisk* 10 moderate	●	20 minutes flat walk 10 brisk 10 moderate	●	20 minutes flat walk 10 brisk 10 moderate	●	20 minutes flat walk 10 brisk 10 moderate
2	20 minutes flat walk all brisk	●	20 minutes flat walk all brisk	●	20 minutes flat walk all brisk	●	20 minutes flat walk all brisk
3	30 minutes flat walk 20 brisk 10 moderate	●	30 minutes flat walk 20 brisk 10 moderate	●	30 minutes flat walk 20 brisk 10 moderate	●	30 minutes flat walk 20 brisk 10 moderate
4	30 minutes flat walk all brisk	●	30 minutes flat walk all brisk	●	30 minutes flat walk all brisk	●	30 minutes flat walk all brisk
5	30 minutes hill walk 15 brisk 15 moderate	●	30 minutes hill walk 15 brisk 15 moderate	●	30 minutes hill walk 15 brisk 15 moderate	●	30 minutes hill walk 15 brisk 15 moderate
6	30 minutes hill walk all brisk	●	30 minutes hill walk all brisk	●	30 minutes hill walk all brisk	●	30 minutes hill walk all brisk

* Brisk is a pace that keeps your heart rate in between 50% and 70% of maximum, as explained on page 68. To improve fitness after Level 6, keep your heart rate towards the upper end, i.e. near 70%.

cycling programme

All the same as the walking programme – a brisk cycling pace will keep your heart rate within the training zone – for people with low or moderate levels of fitness this may be around 8–12 mph; as you get fitter your speed will increase.

NOTE: Find a flat area to cycle in, as uphill work is much harder and downhill work is not aerobic.

swimming programme

Strokes: Vary your strokes – e.g. crawl, breast, back – but always aim to swim at your best pace within your training zone for the allotted time. You can vary your strokes from day to day or within the time periods.

Lengths: Until you complete Level 6, DON'T COUNT LENGTHS as this is a time- and training-zone-based programme, and the amount of lengths you do will depend upon the stroke and your fitness level and strength. – JUST KEEP UP YOUR BEST PACE FOR THE TIMES GIVEN. Once you can swim for 30 continuous minutes within your training-zone heart rate, you can improve further by beginning to count lengths and do more lengths in the same time. This can be achieved by either working harder at the same stroke or changing to a harder stroke.

	day 1	day 2	day 3	day 4	day 5	day 6	day 7
level 1	20 minutes 5 x 3 minutes brisk*, plus l-minute rest between each 3 minute period**	●	20 minutes as day 1	●	20 minutes as day 1	●	●
2	25 minutes 5 x 4 minutes brisk*, plus l-minute rest between each -minute period**	●	25 minutes as day 1	●	25 minutes as day 1	●	●
3	30 minutes 5 x 5 minutes brisk*, plus l-minute rest between each 5-minute period**	●	30 minutes as day 1	●	30 minutes as day 1	●	●
4	33 minutes 3 x 10 minutes brisk*, plus l-minute rest between each 10-minute period**	●	33 minutes as day 1	●	33 minutes as day 1	●	●
5	33 minutes 2 x 15 minutes brisk*, plus l-minute rest between each 15-minute period**	●	33 minutes as day 1	●	33 minutes as day 1	●	●
6	30 minutes non-stop brisk swim	●	30 minutes as day 1	●	30 minutes as day 1	●	●

* Brisk is the fastest you can go while keeping within your training zone. A good test that you are maintaining this is simply that you can keep swimming continuously for the time stated – i.e. 3 minutes for Level 1, 4 minutes for Level 2 , and so on. If you have to stop earlier, swim more slowly and/or use a different stroke.
** Or as long as you need to recover – but if you need more than an extra 30–60 seconds, you are probably swimming too fast and going outside your own training zone.

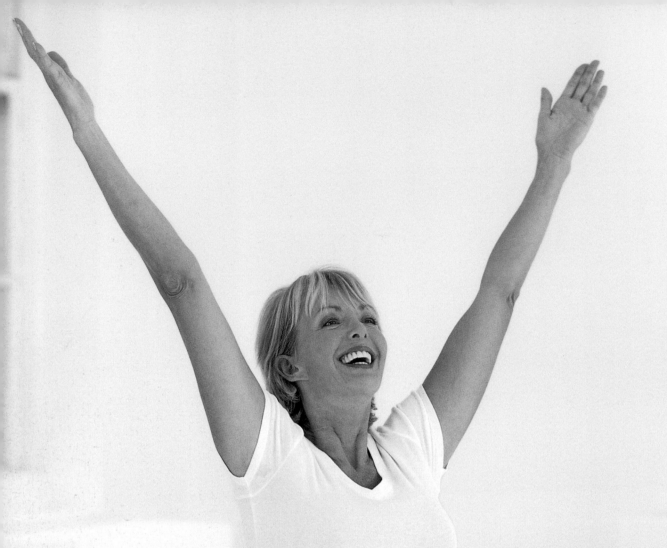

exercise for shape

You may have beautiful skin and no grey hair, but if your body is in bad shape no one will mistake you for someone younger. A poor shape is hard to disguise, instantly ageing and reveals you've been neglecting yourself. More importantly, poor shape is linked with poor health. For example, a fat stomach can be linked with increased risk of heart disease and diabetes. However slim you are, if you don't use your body, you'll lose your shape!

So if you don't like what you see when you look in the mirror before you get dressed in the morning, don't hurriedly turn away, put on those baggy clothes and pretend it was someone else you glimpsed there. All those physical signs of ageing in your appearance can be improved or even removed within months. A simple several-times-a week programme of exercise can re-tone your muscles, realign your body and will smooth out, define and appear to slim down your shape.

why work out?
When we are young, our muscles get plenty of work and have a natural tendency to keep their mass, strength and flexibility. As we begin to age (from around the early 30s onward), however, we need to do some regular work to keep them looking good. And it is our muscle tone that most defines shape and posture – along with supple connecting tissue, which can help prevent muscle imbalance and poor posture.

Research shows that even if you have neglected your muscles and your posture for years, just a few weeks of work can show results. Within around three months, you can lose inches from your waist, redefine your arm and leg muscles, flatten your stomach, firm up your bum, ease back pain and improve flat feet, round shoulders and other posture problems. Even people in their 60s and beyond can improve their shape with exercise.

what to do?
The 10-exercise plan that appears on the next few pages is all that most people will need to give themselves a body with the definition, tone and shape of someone several years younger – or at least the body that YOU had a few years ago!

giveaway signs of a neglected body
Thick waist As both sexes age, their waists tend to thicken, but this is a problem that particularly shows on women – partly because the waist is more defined in young women than it is in men, so the difference is more noticeable as we age, and partly because hormonal changes around the menopause cause women to thicken round the middle. Regular toning and stretching exercises can minimize these effects.

Fat belly Stomach muscles don't naturally get as much exercise as other body parts (e.g. leg muscles used for walking) so they tend to be the first set of muscles to show neglect. As there is nothing to hold the stomach in except muscle, a protruding stomach is a sure sign of poor stomach muscle tone.

Flat bottom Long hours sitting in chairs, cars, etc. soon show in your gluteals – muscles that once gave you a nice rounded bottom. They get elongated and flat – and your bum low-slung, flat and flabby. A few minutes gluteal exercise daily can reverse this.

No tone to limbs This is why women of 50 stop wearing sleeveless tops and skirts above the knee (the pocket of flab just above the knee where there used to be a hollow), and men no longer parade around the pool. Unused bodies lack the undulation of strong smooth muscles. Working out with light weights or your own body weight can give you back a pleasing outline.

General bad posture Years of sitting and standing in lazy or wrong ways give many mid-lifers very poor posture. This shows as rounded shoulders, head poked forward, slightly flat feet, sticky-out belly and shortened waist, and it is often combined with very poor flexibility and range of movement in the joints. Realigning exercises can improve posture tremendously while a few lifestyle changes can make improvement permanent.

the shape programme

The routine here, including warm-up and cool-down, should take you no more than 20 minutes. Do it at least three times a week – four is even better – and you will see real improvement in your shape within weeks. Before you begin, do read all the tips below.

● Exercise in a warm room on a stable mat or towel on carpet. Wear comfortable clothes and lightweight trainers.

● Don't exercise after a heavy meal.

● Read the instructions carefully and look at the illustrations so that you know what you are trying to achieve.

● Do each exercise slowly and steadily, hurrying is counterproductive.

● Breathe normally throughout, unless otherwise instructed.

● If you feel any pain, stop.

● Repeat each move up to 10 times (you may only manage fewer to start with) before resting for 20 seconds and then moving on to the next exercise.

● Don't skip the warm-up – your body will perform better if it is properly warmed and there will be less risk of any muscle strain, pain or injury.

● Don't skip the cool-down stretches. These not only help prevent stiff or sore muscles and maintain muscle elasticity, but also help prevent muscle imbalance.

● Check with your doctor before starting this or any exercise programme.

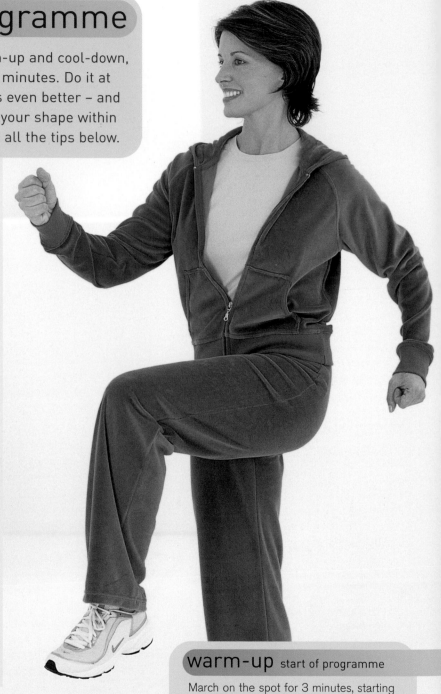

warm-up start of programme

March on the spot for 3 minutes, starting slowly and gently and working up to a more energetic march with the arms swinging and knees lifting higher. For the last 30 seconds, circle your arms. Breathe slowly and deeply throughout.

cool-down end of programme

Do each leg and back stretch described in Exercise for your Weight on pages 82–3, and then add on the following six stretches:

1 gluteal stretch Lie on your back with your knees bent and your feet flat on floor. Cross your right ankle over your left thigh near the knee and bring your legs slowly in towards your chest. Feel the stretch in the right bum area and hip. Hold for a slow count of 10, then return to the starting position and repeat on the other side.

Breathing slowly and deeply can help you to go further into the stretch.

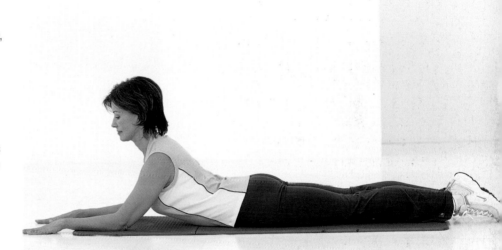

2 lower back stretch From the same starting position as the gluteal stretch, bring both knees in towards your chest, clasping your hands behind your thighs. Feel the stretch in the lower back and hold for a count of 10.

3 abdominal stretch Turn over and lie on your stomach. Bend your arms with your weight on the lower arms, so that your upper body is off the floor as shown. Lift your chest and look ahead of you until you feel a stretch along your abdomen. Hold for a count of 10.

4 chest stretch Sit on the floor and place your hands behind your ears, with your elbows out to your sides. Now gently pull the arms back to feel the stretch across the chest. Hold for a count of 10.

5 shoulder stretch Remain sitting on the floor and bring your right arm across your body. Use your left hand to press gently above the right elbow to bring the right arm in towards your chest, while keeping your right shoulder down. Feel the stretch in your right shoulder. Hold for a count of 10, then repeat with the left arm.

6 side stretch Remain sitting on the floor. Cross your legs and let your left arm support you to the side of your left hip. Bring your right arm up towards the ceiling and over your body until you feel the stretch up your right side. Hold for a count of 10, return to the starting position and repeat on your left side with your right arm supporting.

the shape programme

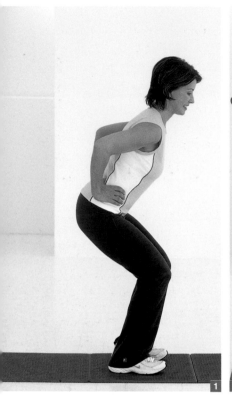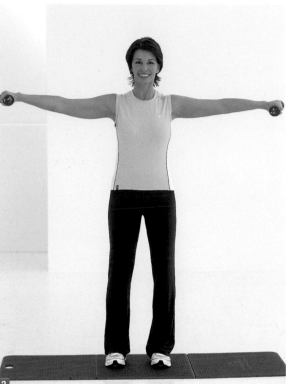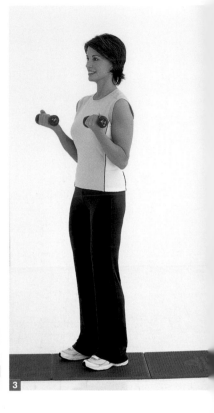

1 parallel squats for the thighs, hips and bottom

Stand with your legs shoulder-width apart, knees relaxed, arms at your sides. Pull the tummy in and tuck the bottom in, your shoulders should be back and down, but keep the posture light, not tight.

Now slowly bend the knees and hips to lower your torso towards the floor, to a maximum of 90 degrees (though you probably won't be able to go that far anyway). Slowly return to standing.

2 lateral arm raises with weights for the shoulders

Take two 1kg weights (or water-filled 750ml bottles) and stand in the starting position (see exercise 1). Have your weights held so that your palms face in to your body. Now slowly raise your arms outwards and upwards until they are at shoulder height, then slowly lower back to the starting position. Remember to keep your stomach stable while doing this exercise, and don't arch your back.

3 bicep curls with weights for the front of the upper arms

Still holding the weights, stand in the same starting position as before. Have your arms in front of you and held down with the palms facing to the front. Now slowly lift your lower arms (from hands to elbows) up and in towards your shoulders and then slowly return to start.

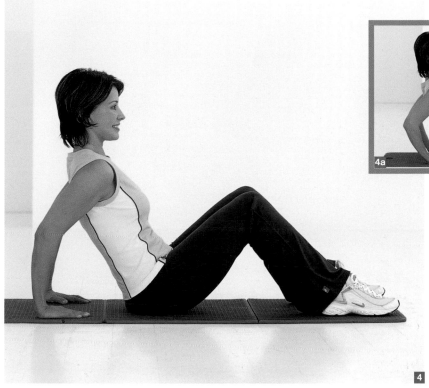

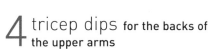

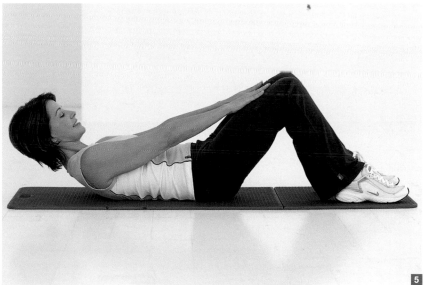

4 tricep dips for the backs of the upper arms

Sit on the floor with your legs bent and upper body slightly back, with the weight supported on your palms placed about 23 cm (9 inches) behind you as shown (4 left). Now bend your elbows and slowly lower your upper body down towards the floor until you are at about 45 degrees (4a above). Slowly return to the starting position.

5 curl-ups abdomen

Lie on the floor on your back with your knees bent, your feet flat on the floor and your arms at your sides. There should be a small gap between your lower back and the floor, but try to keep your stomach tucked in. Lift your head off the floor and, as you do so, very slowly slide your arms towards your knees. Slowly return to the starting position.

NOTE: If this exercise hurts your neck, place a folded towel under your head or consider purchasing an abdominal exerciser cage. In later weeks you can put your hands behind your head to make the curl a little more difficult.

the shape programme

6 diagonal curl-ups for the waist

Start in the same position as for the previous exercise and raise your head and neck off the floor as before, but this time move both arms across your body as if you are trying to reach a point to the side of your right knee. Slowly return to the starting position and repeat to the other side. This counts as one move.

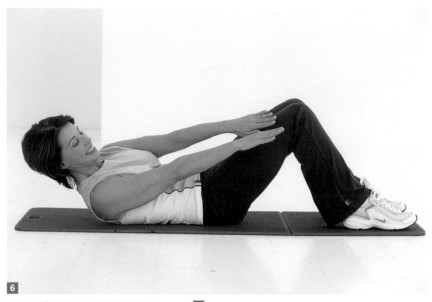

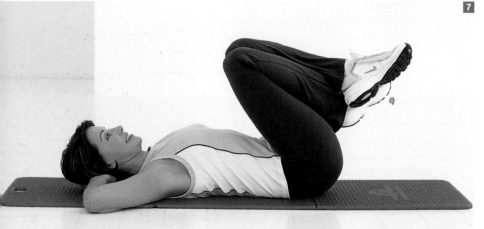

7 double curl-ups for the abdominals

Start in the same position as for the previous exercise. Slowly raise your legs into the air as shown (left), so that your knees are bent and your legs are in towards your chest, then cross your ankles. Now raise your head and neck off the floor (with hands behind your head) and tilt your bottom off the floor a little as you do so (7a). Feel your abdomen working. This is a harder exercise than the previous two, so try only one or two at first and build up gradually. Slowly return to the starting position (but don't place your legs back on the floor until you have completed your reps; just move them back sufficiently to return your bottom to the floor).

8 shoulder raises for the lower back

Turn over on to your stomach, with your legs out straight, although relaxed at the knee. Bend your arms and place your hands under your forehead as shown. Now slowly raise your upper body, head and arms a few inches off the floor, or as far as you can comfortably go, which may be only an inch or so. Slowly return to the starting position. Always keep your legs in contact with the floor and still.

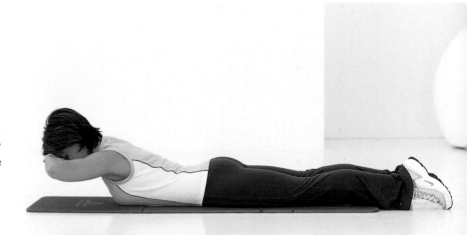

8

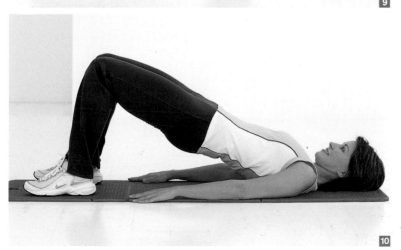

9

9 press-ups for the pectorals (chest) and triceps

Kneel on all fours with your back straight, tummy tucked in, arms under the shoulders and your fingers pointing forward. Now slowly lower your body so that your forehead nearly touches the floor. Slowly return to the starting position.

10 the bridge for the bottom

Lie on your back with your knees bent and your feet flat on the floor, and with your arms at your sides and the palms facing down. Now lift your bottom off the floor slowly until your thighs and body form a diagonal line to the floor. Feel your gluteals working to do this, and keep yourself there for a second before returning slowly to the floor. In later weeks you can hold the position and slowly extend one leg to finish the 'line', then repeat with the other leg.

10

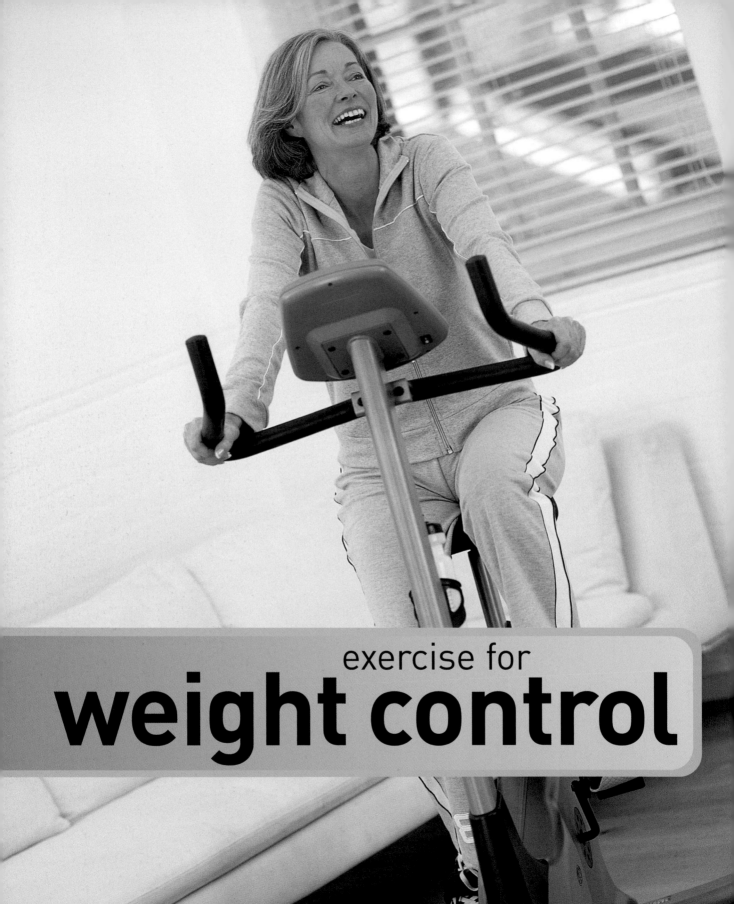

exercise for
weight control

Whether you want to lose weight or simply keep the pounds at bay, the best thing to do is to incorporate regular exercise into your life. This is a simple fact that can't be argued with, as all studies done in recent years show that it is people who keep active who find it easiest to stay slim. And in mid life exercise can be more important than at any other time of your life.

Yet, as we head into our 40s, 50s and 60s, we tend to slow down... often without realizing it. No more competitive sports; no more public transport or walking to work as we get well off enough to take taxis or commute by car; no more cleaning – we can afford to pay someone to do it. And life often is not such a rush – so instead of going everywhere at top speed, we have more time and inclination to dawdle. Just think back to your 20s and early 30s and compare your lifestyle then with now – and I bet you find that you HAVE slowed down. That means you are using fewer calories. A hundred calories a day fewer burnt means a yearly weight gain of about 10 pounds – unless you eat 100 calories a day less to compensate.

The next part of the weight equation is that, in mid life, our natural metabolic rate (MR) begins to slow down, as a part of the general slowing down of the system which carries on until we die. This is true of both sexes, but women experience a particularly marked decline in metabolism around their late 40s and 50s – the menopausal years.

Lastly, the metabolic rate also declines on a par with our loss of muscle. The percentage of muscle (lean tissue) in your body governs, to a large extent, how high or low your metabolic rate is. The more muscle you have, the higher your basal metabolic rate will be (the rate at which you burn calories while doing no work at all – i.e. lying down/sleeping). As we age, we tend to lose muscle steadily.

One study shows that from the ages of 30 to 70, we lose 30% of our lean tissue, which is one reason why younger people have higher MRs than older people. Regular exercise of the right kind can help you to not only hold on to your lean tissue but actually reverse the loss. One US study showed that using resistance (weight-training) programmes, women put on 6kg of lean tissue in 20 weeks, another showed gains of 2.4kg over 10 weeks for men, and all the participants lost body fat as they gained lean tissue.

So what does this mean? In essence, the older you get, the more you need to counteract this metabolic slowdown by taking plenty of calorie-burning exercise (mainly aerobic) and plenty of muscle-conserving exercise (mainly weight-bearing).

Many people ask me, 'Is it possible to lose weight just with exercise alone without changing your eating habits?' The answer is that losing weight just through exercise can be very time-consuming, but it is theoretically possible for a sedentary person to lose about half a pound a week if they begin to exercise regularly. You would need to burn about 1,750 calories to lose half a pound of body fat, i.e. 250 calories extra a day, which roughly translates as an hour's moderate aerobic exercise. That is a simple equation, as it doesn't take account of any increase in your metabolic rate through increasing your lean tissue or making your overall lifestyle more active.

Studies show the best results are achieved with a programme that combines moderate calorie reduction with regular exercise. Once the slimming is over, however, and you just want to maintain weight – then exercise IS definitely your answer. Keep active and you'll keep the surplus pounds off for good.

burning the calories

If you need to lose weight, aim for a minimum of 5–6 exercise sessions a week of sufficient duration that you burn at least 250 calories a session. If you are unfit, however, build up to this level gradually. I suggest you start with any of the programmes - walking, cycling or swimming on pages 70–71. Once you have reached Level 6 on one of those programmes, increase the number and duration of the sessions. If you need to maintain weight, 3–4 sessions a week burning at least 200 calories, should be enough to keep the pounds at bay.

The chart on page 85 shows 30 different ways to burn up 100 and 250 calories, and each activity is star-rated for its lean-tissue-building ability. Before starting any of the activities, check with your doctor that they are suitable for you – particularly if you haven't exercised in some time or have health problems.

In the long term, you should find activities that you enjoy and which fit in with your life, otherwise you won't stick to any plan. Below are some of my own favourite suggestions for aerobic exercise that you might consider. Don't forget to warm up before you begin, cool down in a similar way, and do the cool-down stretches opposite (adding those for the back if you have been swimming). More detailed safety (and other) tips for aerobic exercise appear on page 69.

aerobic exercise

skipping If you are short of time, skipping is one of the best calorie-burning activities. Indeed, unless you are quite fit, to begin with you will find it hard to skip for longer than a minute or two. Do one or two mini-sessions a day (stopping for a few seconds now and then) until you can do several minutes without stopping. As you get more proficient, skip faster or do double jumps (jump twice in the time the rope turns), or try squatting jumps or high knee lifts. You can buy a skipping rope with a built-in calorie-counter. You must wear good training shoes with maximum shock-absorption capacity.

dancing Whether you choose to buy a dance exercise video and prance in front of the TV, go to a dance exercise class or actually go out dancing, exercise to music is one of the activities that is most fun to do. The music helps motivate you and is also very good for your mood, lifting depression and – according to research at Brunel University in London – it can even help you to get fit more quickly by encouraging you to keep going longer and work a bit harder. If you are unfit, choose a beginners' video or class, and progress to fast and furious disco or hip-hop tracks.

'spinning' Much more than just riding an exercise bike at the gym, 'spinning' classes are popular throughout the world now and particularly popular with men. You go for a 'spin' on a stationary mountain bike and can climb steep hills or pedal flat out on the flat. The spin teacher encourages you and you 'spin' to loud techno music. A sixty-minute 'spin' class can burn off more calories than almost any other activity.

1 standing hamstring stretch

Stand with your legs together, then slide the right foot forward and bend your left knee, leaning your body forward and resting your hands on your left thigh as shown. Lean forward from the hips and lift your bottom up, until you feel the stretch up the back of your right thigh. Repeat to the other side.

2 standing lower calf stretch

Stand with your knees slightly bent and your right leg set a few inches behind your left leg as shown. Bend the right knee a little, keeping the heel of the right foot flat on the floor. Feel the stretch in the lower right calf as you do this. Repeat to the other side.

3 standing quad stretch

Stand with your knees relaxed and lift your right leg behind your body as shown, grasping the foot firmly with your right hand. Support yourself with a sturdy chair back if you like. Bring the foot in towards your bottom, keeping the pelvis steady. Feel the stretch up the front of your right thigh. Repeat to the other side.

cool-down stretches hold each stretch for a count of 15

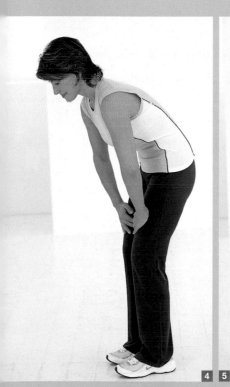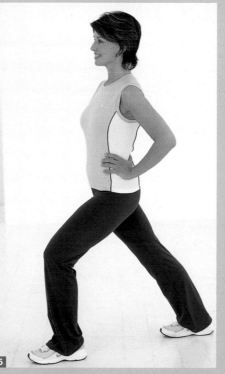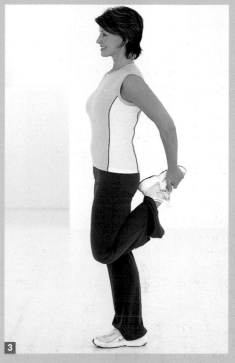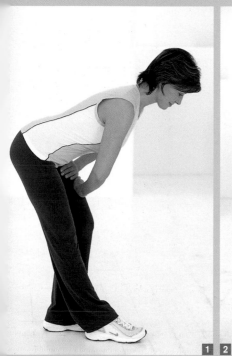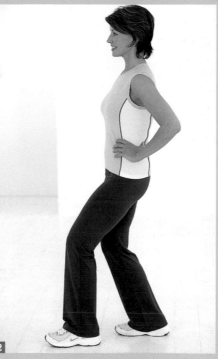

1 2
3
4 5

4 ## standing back stretch

Stand with your feet hip width apart, knees bent and your palms flat on your thighs, fingers facing inwards. Now curve the spine and stretch out your back as shown, feeling your abdomen pulling inwards as you do so.

5 ## upper calf stretch

With the right leg, take a step back about 18 inches and bend your left leg at the knee over your shoe-laces. Keeping the heel on the floor, straighten your right leg and now lean forward slightly and feel a stretch in the upper right calf. Repeat to the other side.

Invest in a pedometer (about £10-20), which will tell you how many steps you take in a day. For weight loss, aim for 10,000 steps a day; for weight control, 5,000 steps a day.

tips for resistance exercise

- If doing resistance training without professional help, follow the instructions that come with your equipment carefully.

- Start off carefully and build up gradually. For free weights, do one set of 8–10 reps for each of the exercises (which should come with the equipment) with a light weight to begin, for example, and then increase the sets and/or reps and/or weight lifted over time.

- Train every other day, or – when you are much stronger – do upper body work one day and lower body work the next day.

- Fewer reps using higher resistance build more lean tissue. More reps using lower resistance are better for toning and endurance.

- Warm up and cool down as for cardiovascular exercise.

- Exercise in a warm room.

- Try to build more resistance work into your everyday life – e.g. carrying shopping bags rather than pushing trolleys.

resistance work

Increasing the percentage of lean tissue (muscle) in your body through resistance exercise is, as we've seen, one of the two major ways of increasing metabolic rate and thus burning calories. Not only that, but resistance work – essentially, working with weights – also helps improve your shape, increases bone density and – looking to the future – will help you retain physical fitness into old age. One research study found that older people who did resistance training found everyday living easier and even walked faster.

As you can see from the Activity Chart opposite, not that many activities actually increase lean tissue by any great amount. Here we look at the ways to get resistance work into your life –one is bound to be right for you.

gym work Today's health clubs and gyms usually offer state-of-the-art variable weight-resistance machines which, properly used, are very safe and suitable for anyone from beginners onwards. Reputable clubs will ensure that you have a resistance programme suitable for your fitness, health and ability, and will give you a fitness assessment and induction before you begin. If you have any health problems, they should also ask for a letter from your doctor.
Pros Top-quality equipment, monitoring, motivation.
Cons Can be expensive, though council-run gyms are not. If you have to travel miles, you may not go as often as you should.

home gym An alternative, which may work out less expensive eventually than health club subscriptions, is to buy equipment for your own home, such as an all-in-one multi-gym or mini-gym. These can vary in price from a few hundred pounds to thousands.
Pros Your are more likely to work out if you don't have to go far.
Cons No one to help you, so the equipment may gather dust unless you are motivated. Space needed.

free weights With a set of dumbbells, a barbell and various weights from 0.5kg up to 4.5kg, you can perform quite a wide range of lean-tissue-building exercises at home.
Pros Inexpensive, can do at home.
Cons No one to help you; free weights may be dangerous if not used correctly. Space needed if using bench.

other small equipment You can buy resistance bands or tubes of different resistance strengths, and achieve similar results to light weights.
Pros Inexpensive, portable (ideal for travelling), little storage space needed.
Cons As you get stronger, this equipment may not offer enough resistance.

body weight If you are very unfit, you can build a certain amount of lean tissue using your body's own weight for resistance. For example, the toning exercises in Exercise for Shape, pages 72–9 could offer a marginal increase in lean tissue.
Pros No equipment needed.
Cons Not as effective as other methods for lean-tissue building.

choosing your activity

NOTE: Always choose an activity that is suitable for your current fitness level. Activities are listed in order of fastest to slowest calorie-burners and figures are approximate. The heavier you are, the more calories you will burn doing the activity. These figures are based on a person weighing 10$\frac{1}{2}$ stones. ● little or no lean-tissue building; ●● builds lean tissue in legs over time, depending on intensity; ●●● good lean-tissue building; ●●●● excellent lean-tissue building.

activity	to burn 100 calories (minutes)	to burn 250 calories (minutes)	lean tissue rating (see above)
squash	7	17.5	●●
spinning	7.3	18.3	●
skipping	9	22.5	●●
stair climbing (or stair machine)	10	25	●●●
swimming, crawl	11	27.5	●
core training	11.2	28	●
circuit training (gym)	12	30	●●●●
jogging	12.5	31.3	●●
kickboxing	13	32.5	●
swimming, breast stroke	13	32.5	●
uphill walking	13	32.5	●●
ashtanga yoga	13.7	34.3	●
horse-riding	14	35	●
tennis	14	35	●
rowing (or machine)	14	35	●●●
badminton	15	37.5	●
cycling, fast	15	37.5	●●
dancing, disco or line	15	37.5	●
digging, heavy	15	37.5	●●
downhill skiing	15	37.5	●
mowing, push-type	15	37.5	●
aerobics class	16	40	●
walking, brisk	16	40	●
golf, average	20	50	●
rollerblading	20	50	●
weight training	21	52.5	●●●●
table tennis	22	55	●
cycling, moderate to slow	25	62.5	●
housework, average	25	62.5	●
bowls	33	82.5	●
dancing, ballroom	33	82.5	●

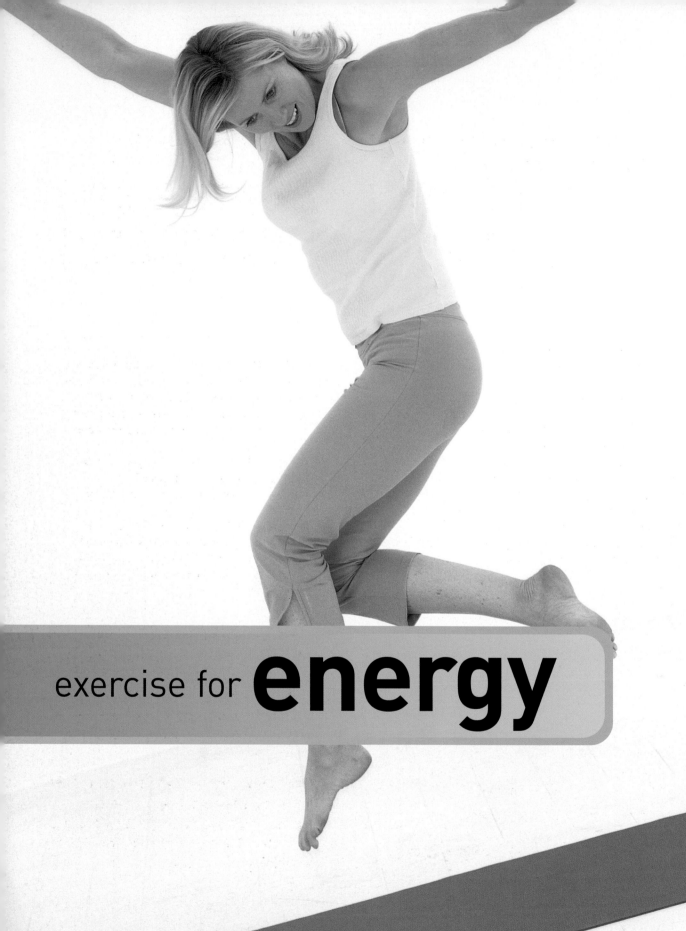

exercise for **energy**

If you are one of those people who equates exercise with tiredness, fatigue and the urgent need to lie down, you'll be wondering how it can actually energize you. Tackled in the right way, however, indeed it can. Exercise can sometimes be better than sleep for helping you to feel fresh and lively. It can be a big boost for both mental and physical energy, and can help revamp your sex life and your sleep patterns.

To be energizing, exercise doesn't always have to be energetic — although sometimes it can be. Here are the ways in which exercise energizes.

banishing tiredness
Exercise — particularly aerobic exercise (which gets the heart beating faster and the lungs breathing in more deeply) — speeds the circulation of blood around the body and delivers more oxygen to the brain and muscles — indeed, to all parts of the body. This has the effect of revitalization and is especially good at alleviating 'brain tiredness' or feelings of tiredness that seem to come on for little reason during the day, or after a carbohydrate meal. Exercising outdoors, in cool air, also has a refreshing and revitalizing effect.

increasing alertness and mental energy
Research shows regular exercise improves mental stamina and energy. It may do this by increasing the amount of blood and oxygen — and therefore nutrients — that reaches the brain. Exercise speeds up the metabolic rate and appears to increase brain activity — speeding up thought processes and giving you a sharpness that shows in faster speech and more lucid expression. Because exercise lifts depression, it can clear the mental 'fog' that makes depressed people seem slow to react. Canadian research shows that depressed people improve with as little as 20 minutes' exercise 3 times a week. Exercise makes us breathe more deeply, which in turn calms us and helps us feel more self-confident, improving performance.

increasing strength
Resistance exercise (see pages 84–5) helps strengthen and build lean tissue. Increased strength means you can work longer, and harder, at all physical activities and this can help to prevent physical tiredness.

reviving sexual energy
Improved circulation and strength can help revive libido and improve sexual performance. One cause of impotence in males is a diminished blood supply to the penis, for example. And female sexual sensitivity is enhanced with improved blood supply to the vaginal area.

improving quality of sleep
If you exercise regularly, research shows your quality of sleep improves — you sleep more deeply, more soundly and wake more refreshed.

stimulating hormones
Exercise can release hormones, such as dopamine and serotonin, which can lift depression, banish the feelings of lethargy and fatigue that depression often brings, and produce a sense of well-being sometimes known as the 'exercise high'.

▶ **don't over-exercise** Doing too much, too soon, or overtaxing your muscles or heart and lungs WILL make you feel tired. The best exercise for energy is moderate and is something that you enjoy.

don't exercise when you are genuinely tired For example, if you have been up for 18 consecutive hours without sleep, it will be better to go to bed than start exercising to try to find energy.

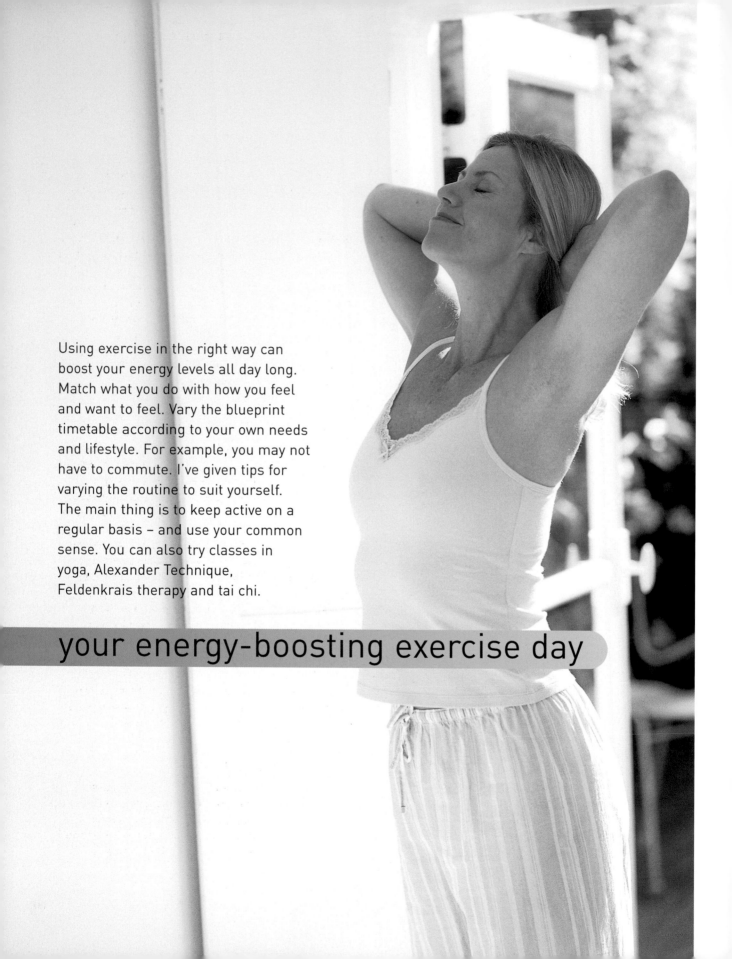

Using exercise in the right way can boost your energy levels all day long. Match what you do with how you feel and want to feel. Vary the blueprint timetable according to your own needs and lifestyle. For example, you may not have to commute. I've given tips for varying the routine to suit yourself. The main thing is to keep active on a regular basis – and use your common sense. You can also try classes in yoga, Alexander Technique, Feldenkrais therapy and tai chi.

your energy-boosting exercise day

7 am – on waking

If you've slept with an open window you shouldn't feel too sluggish – but now is a good time to go over to that window and do some deep breathing to get oxygen circulating around your body. Couple it with some shoulder shrugs and small arm circles, and within a minute or two you should feel wide awake.

Any stiffness from the night? Arch your back (see warm-up exercises on page 74) and slowly and gently bring your head down first to your right shoulder and then up and over to your left, looking forward all the time.

8.30 am – journey to work

After a small healthy breakfast, if possible build some exercise into your morning commute. Even if you can't walk or cycle all the way, perhaps you can walk to the next bus or train stop instead of the nearest one, or get off at a stop further away from work. If you drive in to work, could you park a bit further away?

Even 15 minutes' walking in the morning will get your heart rate up, improve your circulation and help burn off calories, and will boost brain power so that you work better. If you have any stress about work, the walk will also help you to relax.

tips ● If you don't commute, build in a never-to-be-missed 15–30 minutes to get out of your home and bring your body to life with some exercise.
● Don't try to do hard aerobic or resistance work too early in the morning – most people's bodies can't cope at this time; wait until early evening if possible.

11.30 am – break time

After a few hours at work, you may be feeling stressed out mentally, as morning is when most pressure is on. Use a 10-minute break to have a change of scene – walk up a few flights to take in a view from the roof terrace; walk down to the grounds or, if that isn't possible, do some stretches in the stockroom or boardroom. No one should go more than 2–3 hours sitting or standing in the same place without a break. A banana and a cup of tea make ideal break-time snack food.

tip ● If you are at home, you too should take a break from whatever you're doing. A few minutes on a rebounder would be a good pick-you-up.

1.30 pm – lunch

Take at least a 20-minute walk before your lunch and incorporate some deep breathing (see pages 110–11). Make lunch high in protein and low in carbs, so you don't suffer a slump in the afternoon.

tip ● If your schedule means that you have to go to the gym or a class in your lunch break, skip workout time later.

3 pm – afternoon break

By now you may be feeling a bit stiff around the shoulders, neck or lower back and generally a bit tired or tense, especially if you work at a desk or do a lot of driving or standing for long hours. You need to do five minutes' stretching to suit your own problem areas (see stretches on pages 82–3). Relax your face with some forced yawns and cup your hands over your eyes to ease eye strain. A green tea and an apple will complete your quick afternoon re-energizer.

6.30 pm – workout time

Research shows that around 6–7pm is the best time to ask your body to do formal exercise – such as gym work, an exercise class or a workout video in front of the TV. So rather than rushing home to a gin and tonic, use the gym as your tonic! If you're planning to do the workouts in this book, now is the time. Follow them with an invigorating shower before supper time. Don't leave aerobic or resistance training any later than 8pm, otherwise you may not sleep well.

tip ● If your working hours carry on until 7pm or so, try to do your workout before you commute home.

10 pm – winding down

Now you need wind-down exercise to help you sleep well. Yoga and/or stretching are ideal, but you don't need to do more than 10–15 minutes.

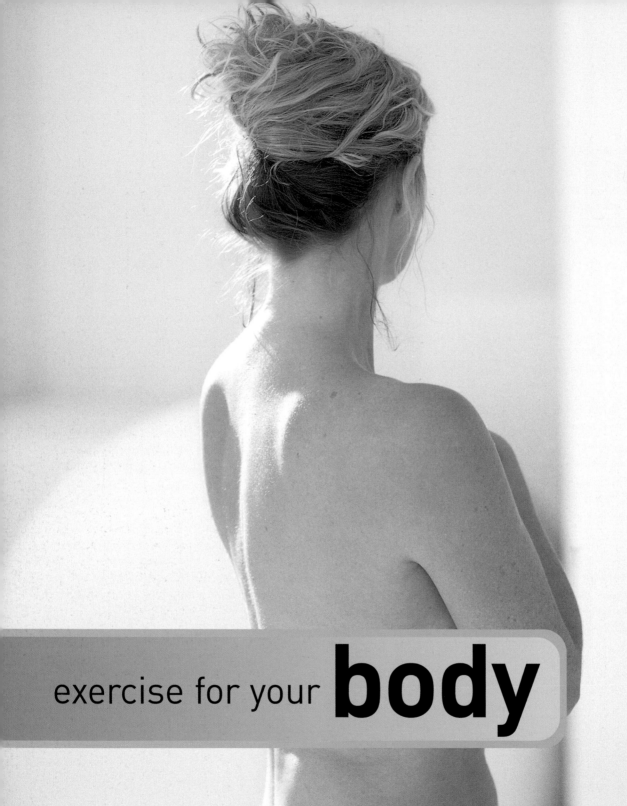

exercise for your **body**

As we move out of young adulthood into so-called 'middle age', one of the most shocking things that can happen to us – worse even than the first sighting of a wrinkle or grey hair – is the realization that we have 'aches and pains'. For years we sail through life mistreating our bodies and taking them for granted and now, suddenly – or so it seems – the body is paying us back... back pain, joint pain, neck pain, hip pain, knee pain ...

Even if there isn't a lot of pain as such, we may find that we can't quite reach or stretch or twist or run quite as well as we used to. Or that there is a certain stiffness in the back or hips after a few hours in bed, or that joints sprain more easily than they used to.

The fact is that a sedentary lifestyle causes – or makes worse – most of these complaints and symptoms, and that regular activity can keep almost any body in good working order and largely free from the disabilities that signal the end of youth. But it is never too late to reverse these symptoms. In one study in the USA of residents of a nursing home with an average age of 87, just 10 weeks' training of $2^{1}/_{4}$ hours a week improved their strength, fitness, gait, balance and speed by up to 100%.

In the next few pages, we look at how exercise can minimize back, joint and muscular aches and pains, and help to prevent the bone degeneration that can lead to osteoporosis.

back pain In the UK alone, back pain costs approximately £5-6 billion a year in health costs and lost manpower. Over 10 million working days are lost each year because of it, and nearly 50% of the adult population regularly suffers from some kind of back pain. And yet many back problems are preventable if we do some simple daily exercises and keep active, and most bad backs can be 'cured' with similarly simple remedial exercises.

arthritis and stiff joints It is now believed that osteoarthritis pain can be minimized with exercise, and that age-associated stiffness is often a result of inactivity and inflexibility in the joints.

rheumatism and fibromyalgia According to scientific research, muscular aches and random pains that may be sporadic, acute or chronic, and are often included under the umbrella of rheumatism or fibromyalgia, can be significantly improved with regular exercise.

osteoporosis The loss of bone density which can lead to osteoporosis can be minimized with regular exercise. Although bone loss doesn't cause pain in its initial stages, and may be hard to detect without a proper scan, in later middle age and old age it can cause fractures, skeletal shrinking and misalignment, and considerable incapacity – so it is well worth beginning a bone maintenance programme as soon as possible.

exercises for your back

The routine here, including warm-up and cool-down, should take you no more than 20 minutes. Do it at least 3 times a week – 4 is even better – and you will see real improvement in your shape within weeks. Before you begin, do read all the tips below.

In recent years there has been a big change in the way experts suggest that we manage back pain. Bed rest used to be prescribed, but staying in bed for days usually serves only to weaken the muscles that support the back even further, and stiffens the whole body. In most cases, this only makes your back worse, while keeping active and following the right kind of exercise plan can reduce pain and increase mobility.

Most acute back pain is caused when a muscle or ligament is pulled via sudden overuse – very common in mid life, as we tend to use our backs only infrequently, which makes them weak, and then do something like very heavy lifting or digging, or even just twisting into an unusual position – e.g. to reach something.

Then there is 'wear and tear' back pain, caused by the discs in the spine becoming less flexible, thinner and less able to absorb shock. This can cause the vertebrae to move closer together, and this in turn causes pain and strain. Also you can have a 'slipped disc', when one or more discs press on the nerves that run along the length of the spine, which also causes pain. Adequate fluid and fatty acid intake (see Section 1) and regular exercise to preserve back and abdominal muscles will help prevent the pain of 'wear and tear' by offering support and stability; stretching exercises help maintain back flexibility, which is often very poor in older adults, and also help to release muscle tension, which can cause chronic long-term back pain. Exercise can also maintain bone density, which helps preserve the spine and prevent pain.

For what to do during an acute attack of back pain, see opposite. For maintaining your back in good condition, and thus helping prevent recurring back pain, try the exercises on the following pages.

look at your lifestyle

To help prevent or minimize back pain, use the following tips in everyday life:

- When carrying, try to distribute weight evenly in both hands.

- When lifting, bend at the knees, keep the abdominals tight and the feet wide apart, and lift the object keeping it as close to your body as you can.

- When sitting, don't slump in the chair. Try to use chairs which have a depth that matches your upper leg length, as well as a supportive back.

- Use a good mattress – medium-firm suits most people – and use only one pillow.

- Evidence suggests that there is an emotional component with much back pain.

- Anxiety, depression and stress can all make pain worse. Research reported in the *Journal of Industrial Medicine* found that people who were unhappy at work or who had to work at pressure were more likely to feel back pain than other people.

helpful tools for a bad back

- A wooden backstretcher (widely available) which you lie on, on the floor, can help improve posture and posture-related back problems.

- Chiropractors and osteopaths are recognized as being able to help maintain a healthy back by manipulation and massage. They are excellent for restoring an acute back to the non-painful stage.

- Deep-tissue massage (e.g. Swedish, physiotherapy) can relieve back pain by aiding relaxation.

- Acupuncture can help acute back pain where other methods have failed or can't be used.

acute back pain

- First apply to the painful area an ice pack or frozen peas covered with a tea towel. This will help reduce inflammation.

- Then applying warmth (e.g. a hot water bottle) to the surrounding area will help the surrounding muscles – which may have gone into spasm to try to protect the area – to relax.

- Painkillers taken in the first 24 hours of bad back pain will also help the muscles to come out of spasm and thus get you out of the common spiral when you feel pain and then tense up even more because of it.

- Rest on your back for a few hours if necessary and, while you do so, try exercises 1 and 2 on the next page regularly to ease the pain.

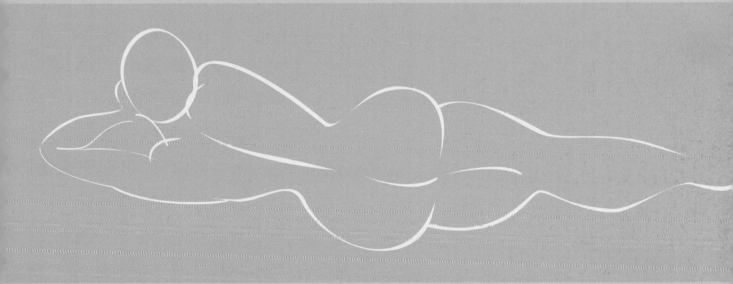

- When the pain moves from 'pain' to the lesser category of 'ache', begin exercises 3 and 4 on page 95 and try to move around as much as you can, without twisting or sudden movements.

- See your doctor for advice if your back pain is no better in 24 hours – and if it was caused by a fall or other obvious injury, if you have trouble passing urine, if you have pain or numbness in your legs or the pain worsens.

- Do regular back exercises (5–9 on the following pages, the stretches on pages 75, 82–3, and abdominal exercises on pages 77–8). Keep active to prevent future attacks.

- The exercises for your joints, bones and relaxation are also relevant (see pages 98–107 and 112–13).

exercise for your back

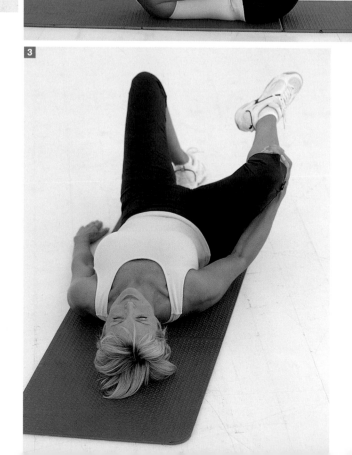

2 the rock

Start from the same position as exercise 1, but, as you bring your knees in to your chest, lift your neck slightly and rock slowly back and forth, massaging your spine with the movement. NOTE: This is for lower back pain – if you have neck pain, stick to exercise 1.

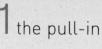

1 the pull-in

Lie on your back (on a comfortable floor or your bed) with your knees bent in towards your chest. Clasp your knees just below the joint around the front, as shown, and relax. Now gently pull both knees in further towards your chest and feel the stretch in your lower back. Relax and repeat several times, several times a day.

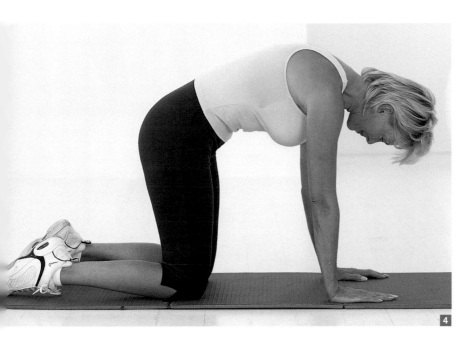

4 back arch

Kneel on all fours on the floor with your hands shoulder-width apart. Look down at the floor as you arch your back, breathing out and pulling your stomach in as you do so. Now slowly lower your stomach towards the floor, breathing in and hollowing your back slightly, and look up to the ceiling.

5 walking hands

Kneel on all fours on the floor with your hands shoulder-width apart. Now, without any sudden twisting movements, slowly 'walk' your hands around to the right side as far as you can without undue strain. Then slowly walk them back to centre and then around to the left side. Repeat 10 times.

3 hip rotation

Lie on your back on a comfortable floor or your bed, with your knees bent and your feet flat on the floor/bed. Now lift your right foot from the floor and in a few inches towards your chest, clasping your hand around the knee as in exercise 1. Keeping your left foot firmly on the bed/floor and your left leg still, gently rotate the right knee clockwise to rotate the right hip. Do this 10 times, then rotate anticlockwise, and repeat with the left leg.

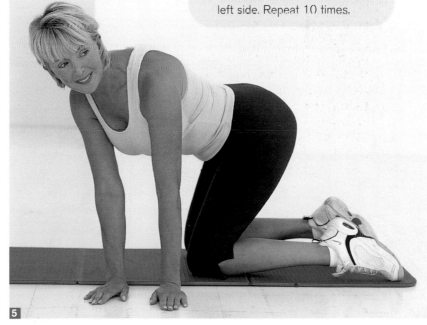

exercise for your back

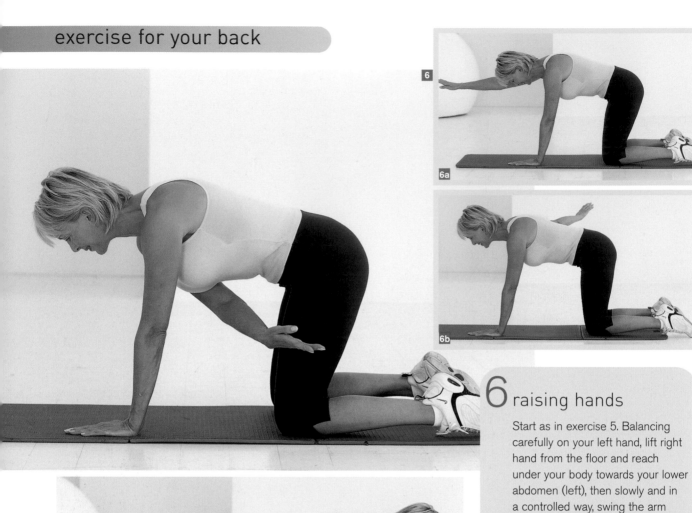

6 raising hands

Start as in exercise 5. Balancing carefully on your left hand, lift right hand from the floor and reach under your body towards your lower abdomen (left), then slowly and in a controlled way, swing the arm out to your right side (with the arm straight but loose at the elbow), following the movement with your eyes, and return it to starting position (6a and b). Repeat with the left hand.

7 knee raises

Start as in exercise 6. Now, balancing carefully on your left knee, lift your right knee up and aim to touch your left elbow — just going as far as you can without undue strain. Return to the starting position and repeat up to 10 times, then repeat with your left knee.

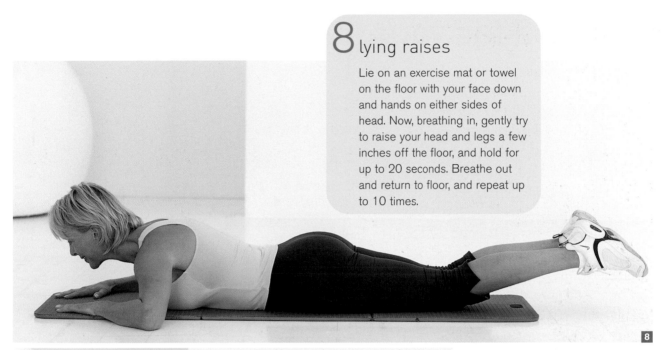

8 lying raises

Lie on an exercise mat or towel on the floor with your face down and hands on either sides of head. Now, breathing in, gently try to raise your head and legs a few inches off the floor, and hold for up to 20 seconds. Breathe out and return to floor, and repeat up to 10 times.

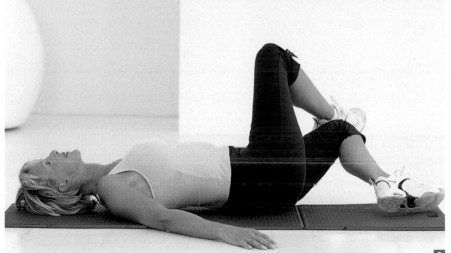

9 lying hip and bum stretch

Lie on the floor on your back with your knees bent and feet flat on the floor, hip-width apart. Now bring your right foot off the floor and in to rest on the top of the left thigh near the knee. Then move your left leg slowly down to the side so that your left knee touches the floor (or as near as you can get without undue strain), as shown. As you go, you will feel a stretch across your right hip and bottom – the more the feel of the stretch, the tighter your bum and hips are. This is a common cause of low back pain. Hold for a count of up to 20, then return to the starting position and repeat to the other side.

other exercise to try...

pilates Concentrates on improving abdominal strength and flexibility, and thus improves posture and back strength.

alexander technique Helps improve posture and relaxation, and helps the back to work with minimum strain on the spine.

gyrotonics Similar to pilates but with more emphasis on three-dimensional movement, which may be ideal for back maintenance rather than beginner's work.

yoga Improves flexibility, posture and relaxation, and may improve strength too. (See pages 112–13 for more on yoga.)

exercise for your joints

If your joints are painful or stiff, or ache from time to time, you need to do regular flexibility work. Arthritis can also be helped with gentle exercise. If you have rheumatoid arthritis, it is best to rest when you have a flare-up and exercise at other times. Research shows the best treatment for osteoarthritis is not to avoid exercise, as many do, but to keep as active as you can. And, if you have muscular aches and pains (often termed fibromyalgia if severe), you will benefit from keeping active (see below). For anyone with stiffness and/or muscular aches or pains, it will help if you have a warm bath before exercise, if you take regular omega-3 fish oils, and if you exercise in a warm room when feeling relaxed. Warm yourself up further by a little marching on the spot, with small arm circles, before you begin. If in doubt, first see your doctor.

fibromyalgia

Chronic muscular/skeletal pain with no medical cause affects about 13% of people in the UK, and often begins in the 40s or 50s. When it is severe it is termed fibromyalgia. Recent research published in the *British Medical Journal* found that graded low-impact (walking and cycling) aerobic exercise gave significant benefits lasting for up to 12 months in those who completed the programme over three months. The Level 1 walking and cycling programmes on page 70 would be suitable for most sufferers. Relaxation and stretching exercises have also been shown to have benefit.

1

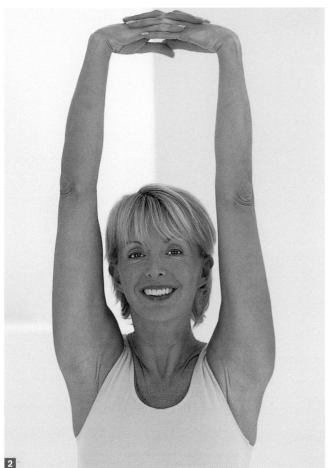

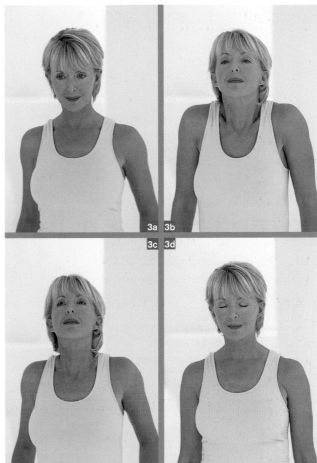

1 neck release Good for relieving neck pain and releasing tension

Sit in a supportive office or kitchen chair and relax your shoulders as much as you can. Bring your head sideways down to the left, looking forward and without twisting your head. Now raise your left arm up and over your head and place the palm of your left hand on the right side of your head. Use moderate pressure to bring your head a little lower down towards your left shoulder. Hold for a count of 10, then return to the starting position and repeat to the other side.

2 shoulder release Good for tense and stiff shoulders

Sit as in exercise 1 and lock your fingers together in front of you so that your palms face downwards. Now extend your arms out in front of you, still with fingers locked, and then on upwards until your arms are over your head (or as far as you can get). When you reach the furthest point that is comfortable, hold for a count of 10–20, then slowly return to the starting position.

3 shoulder rolling Good for tense and stiff shoulders.

Sit as in exercises 1 and 2, with your shoulders down and as relaxed as possible (3a), palms in your lap. Keeping the neck and arms still, raise the shoulders straight up until they are near your ears (3b), then move them backwards (3c) and finally down to the starting position. Do 10 slow rolls and then repeat, moving your shoulders back first (3d) before moving them up and then back to the starting position.

exercise for your joints

4 wrist flexibility Good for stiff, weak or aching wrists

Sit or stand, keeping your elbows at your sides, and bend each arm so that the forearms are out in front of you, palms down. Keeping the arms still, raise your hands from the wrist up as far as they will go (4a). Repeat 5 times, then, with the wrists flat, move your forearms round so that your palms face upwards, then smoothly move them back. Repeat 10 times. Lastly, hold your forearms so that your palms face inwards, fingers loosely bent, and bring hands in towards your chest without moving your arms (4b), feeling the stretch across the back of each wrist. Repeat 10 times.

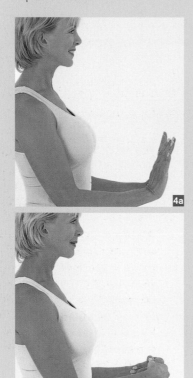

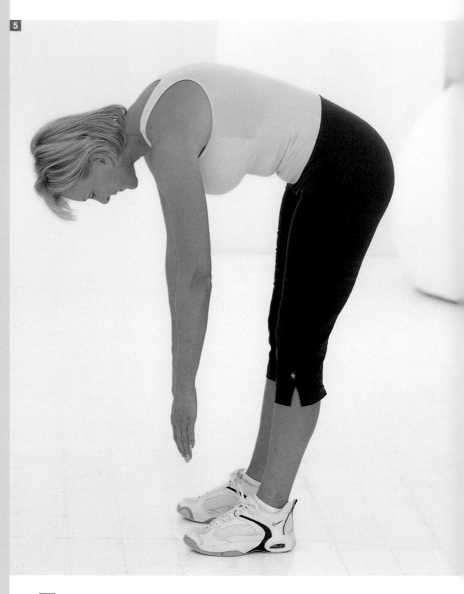

5 standing curl downs Good for relaxing and loosening the spine

Stand against a wall, with the backs of your heels about 3 inches from the wall and your back flat against the wall (or as flat as it will go, keeping a small hollow in the lower spine). Now tighten the abdominal muscles slightly and slowly curl your upper body down until all your spine is away from the wall except the tail-bone. Hang loosely for 10 seconds, then slowly curl back up again, using your stomach muscles to help you.

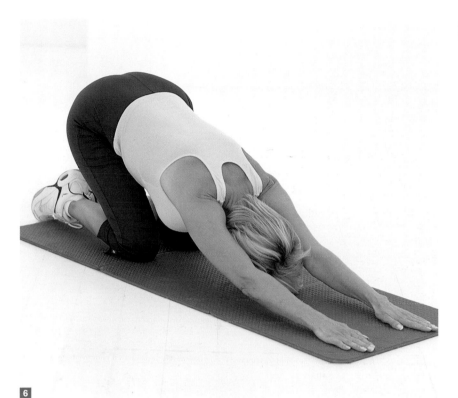

6

6 long back stretch Good for stretching the muscles of the shoulders and back, and releasing the vertebrae of the spine and neck

Kneel on a mat on all fours and slowly slide your bottom back on to your heels, sliding your arms forward and keeping your head tucked in as you do so. When your arms are fully stretched and form a line with your spine, hold for a count of 10 (work this up to 30 as you get used to it). Using the abdominal muscles, slowly come up from the position to a kneel with your arms in the air. Bring your arms down to your sides.

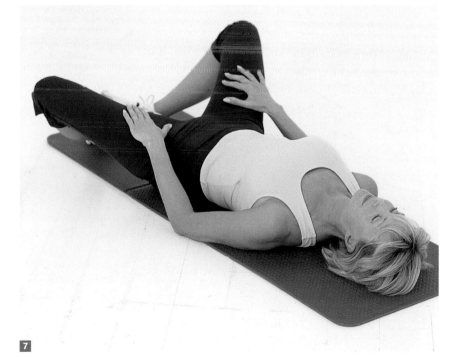

7

7 groin stretch Good for tight pelvic and inner thigh area

Lie on a mat on your back (with your head supported by a cushion if you like), hands resting lightly on your chest. Bring your feet in towards your pelvis, soles facing each other so that your bent legs drop down and out to either side. When they have dropped as far as they will, place each palm flat on your inner thigh near the knee and gently push the legs down a little lower, aiming to keep your spine from arching. When you feel a stretch along the inner thigh, hold for 10, then release.

exercise for your joints

8 lying lower back stretch Good for freeing up a tight lower back

Lie on a mat on your back (with your head supported by a cushion if you like), your arms out to the sides. Now, with your head inclined to the left and the left arm flat on the floor throughout, lift your left leg, with knee bent, up and over to your right side so that your left foot is level with your right knee and your left knee drops down towards the floor. Place your right palm on your left knee and gently exert pressure so that the knee moves a little closer to the floor. Feel a stretch across your lower back and hold for a count of 10. Slowly return to the starting position and repeat to the other side.

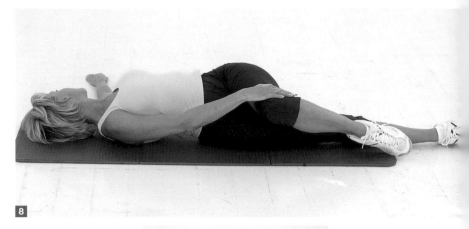

9 hip flex Good for stretching out the large muscles that control hip movement and are often tight, which can cause knock-on pain throughout the lower body

Stand with your arms by your sides and your feet hip-width apart. Now bring your left leg forward and bend at the knee until your knee is over your ankle. As you do so, take your right leg back so that you are in a lunge position, with the right heel slightly off the floor. Now press your pelvis down towards the floor (dropping your right knee slightly to achieve this) so that you feel the stretch along the front of the right hip. Hold for a count of 10, then slowly return to the starting position and repeat to the other side.

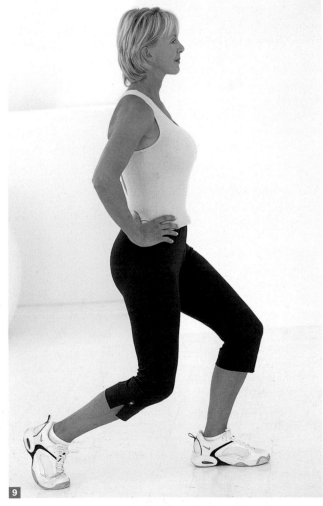

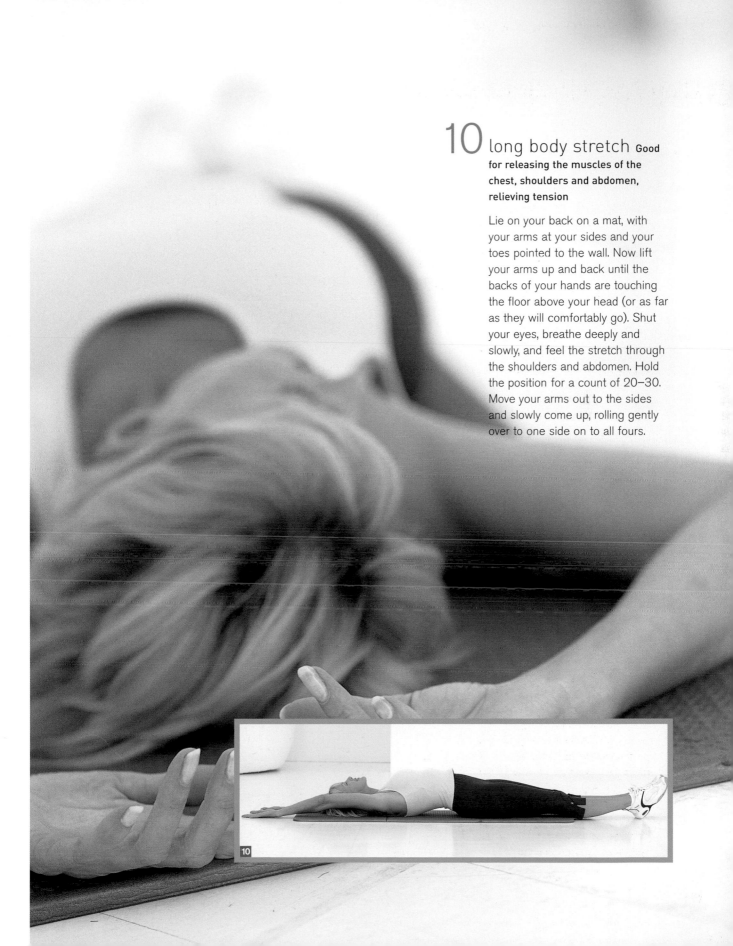

10 long body stretch

Good for releasing the muscles of the chest, shoulders and abdomen, relieving tension

Lie on your back on a mat, with your arms at your sides and your toes pointed to the wall. Now lift your arms up and back until the backs of your hands are touching the floor above your head (or as far as they will comfortably go). Shut your eyes, breathe deeply and slowly, and feel the stretch through the shoulders and abdomen. Hold the position for a count of 20–30. Move your arms out to the sides and slowly come up, rolling gently over to one side on to all fours.

10

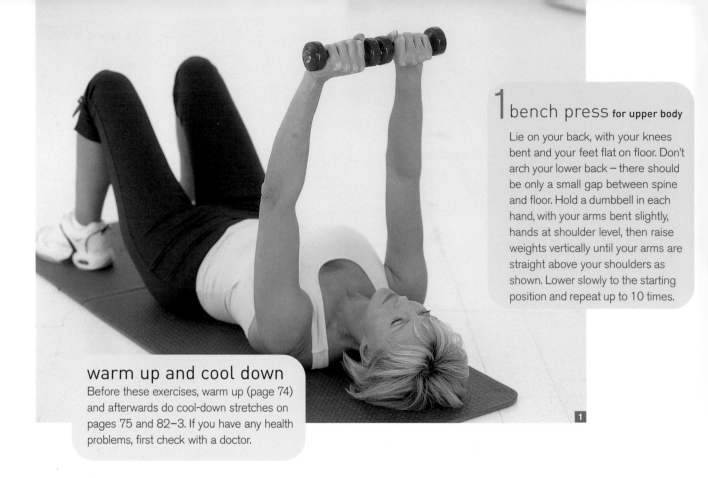

1 bench press for upper body

Lie on your back, with your knees bent and your feet flat on floor. Don't arch your lower back – there should be only a small gap between spine and floor. Hold a dumbbell in each hand, with your arms bent slightly, hands at shoulder level, then raise weights vertically until your arms are straight above your shoulders as shown. Lower slowly to the starting position and repeat up to 10 times.

warm up and cool down

Before these exercises, warm up (page 74) and afterwards do cool-down stretches on pages 75 and 82–3. If you have any health problems, first check with a doctor.

exercise for your bones
Although osteoporosis doesn't usually make itself known until you are in your 60s or later, the process of bone demineralization can begin as early as in the 20s or 30s. It is believed that osteopenia (early bone loss) is suffered by 16% of white women in their 20s.

The most important alterable controlling factor in bone density is regular bone-loading (weight-bearing) exercise, which can be obtained via some forms of aerobic exercise and by using either free weights or your own body weight to provide resistance.

aerobic exercise
Skipping and on-the-spot jumping are two good simple bone-loaders for the lower body and can take only 2–3 minutes a day. If you suffer from arthritis or have been advised not to jar your joints (say, if you already have osteoporosis), then you can instead use a rebounder – a mini-trampoline. Jogging, running and walking (see page 70) are also lower-body bone-loaders, but cycling and swimming are not as your weight is borne by the cycle or the water. The only upper-body bone-loading aerobic exercise commonly available is rowing.

weighted exercise
Research published in the *Journal of the American Medical Association* showed that strength training just twice a week cuts risk of bone fractures in older women. This appears to work because when the muscles contract during the resistance stage they pull against the bones, which in turn stimulates them to grow. Because most aerobic exercise is useful only for the bones in the legs, you should try to do weighted work to stimulate bone repair and renewal in your upper body.

The six examples that follow show bone-building exercises that rely either on free weights or your own body weight to work. The exercises cover the shoulders and arms, spine, hips, and legs, and you will need a pair of 1–2 kg dumbbells to do them.. Do them every day, or at least 3–4 times a week.

2 press-ups for upper body and arms

Kneel on the floor on all fours with hands hip-width apart and feet crossed and raised off the floor, as shown. Keeping the abdominals strong, bend your elbows and slowly lower your upper body down towards the floor, touching the floor with your forehead. Slowly rise again and repeat 10 times.

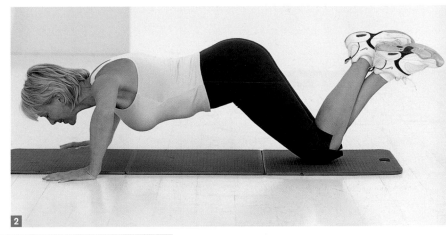

3 seated curls for wrists and forearms

Sit on the edge of a sturdy chair or bench with your legs apart, as shown. Rest your left elbow on your left knee and hold a dumbbell in your right hand with your right arm extended to the floor and the right elbow touching the inside of the right knee as shown (3). Now curl the right forearm up to bring the weight towards the left side of your chest as shown (3a), hold for a count of 2, then slowly return to the starting position. Repeat 10 times and then repeat to the other side.

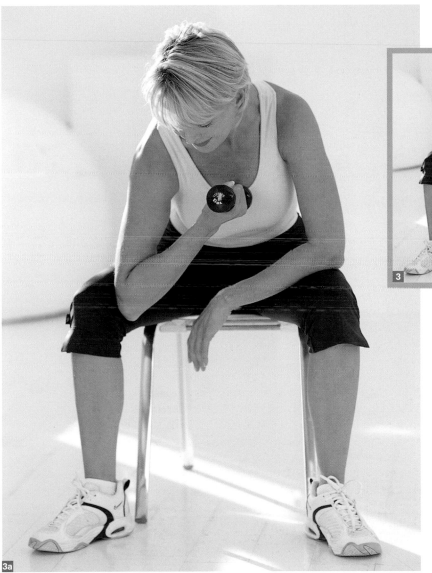

exercise for your bones

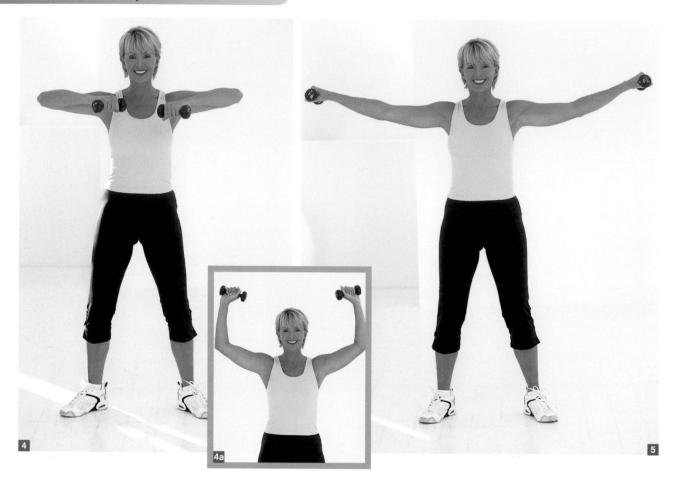

4 shoulder press
for shoulders and arms

Stand with feet hip-width apart and your feet firmly on the floor a few inches apart. Hold the dumbbells with your arms bent at either side of your shoulders, palms facing downward. (4) Now extend your arms upwards above your shoulders (4a), hold for a count of 2, then slowly return to the starting position and repeat 10 times.

5 standing lateral raises
for shoulders and upper back

Stand with feet hip-width apart and a dumbbell in each hand by your sides, palms facing inwards. Now breathe in and slowly raise the dumbbells out to either side of your body, keeping the arms straight, until the dumbbells are slightly above shoulder height. Hold for a count of 2, then slowly return to starting position and repeat 10 times.

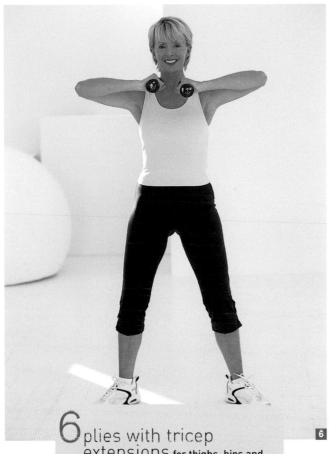

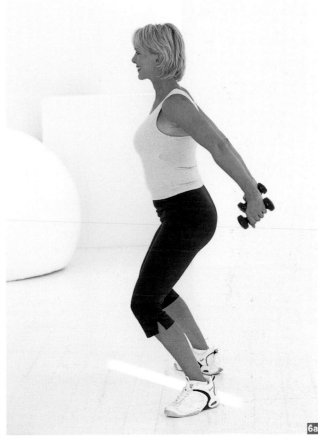

6 plies with tricep extensions for thighs, hips and upper arms

Stand with legs further than hip-width apart, toes pointing out to 45 degrees and a dumbbell in each hand. Keeping abdominals strong throughout, raise elbows, palms towards floor, knuckles facing each other, so upper arms are parallel to floor and out to the sides as shown (6). Keeping feet flat on the floor and chest up, bend knees and lower body until thighs are parallel to floor (or as far as you can comfortably go). As you do so, bring arms out to sides and behind body as far as they will comfortably go (6a). Slowly raise yourself up again and return arms to raised starting position. Repeat 10 times.

are you at risk?

Some people are more prone to osteoporosis than others. Check the list and see if you may have a higher risk factor.

Female ● Post-menopausal ● Tall ● Body Mass Index under 19 ● Parent suffers from osteoporosis ● Caucasian or Asian ● Late onset of menstrual periods ● Early menopause ● Steroids, thyroid treatment or some other medications.

If you think you have a high risk factor, you can get a DXA scan, usually available on the NHS if you are 'at risk', or privately.

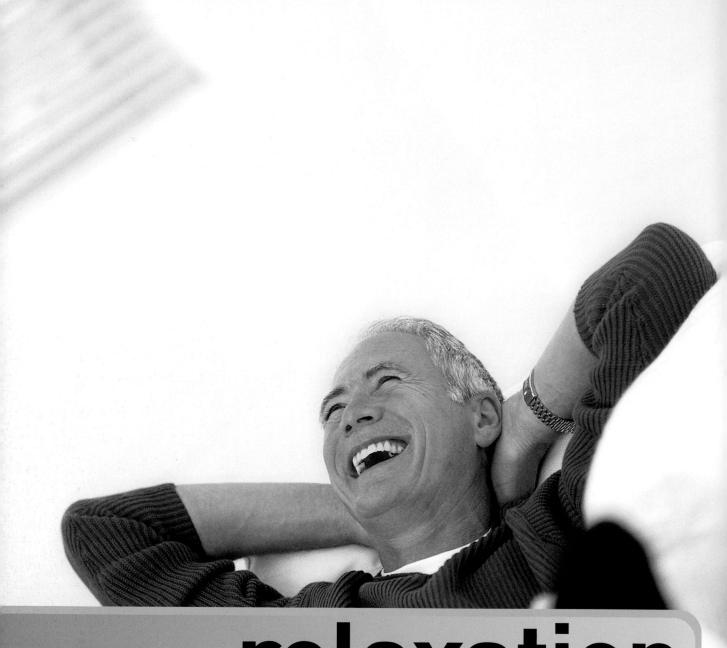

exercise for **relaxation**

What relaxes your mind tends also to relax your body, and vice versa – and exercise is one of the great ways of achieving both mental and physical destressing.

Just as it is hard to separate the relaxation of your mind and your body – the two nearly always go together – when you exercise with relaxation as your goal, you will nearly always find yourself re-energized and less tired too.

This is because stress is one of the great energy-sappers, and if you replace it with calmness, the stress gap is usually soon filled with energy. So exercise for relaxation has much more benefit than you might at first imagine.

The foundation of true relaxation is the ability to breathe properly, a talent which few of us have, or even think about – and even fewer would ever consider to be 'real' exercise. So overleaf we look at this neglected function and find out just why it is important. The simple but vital breathing exercises will help you to breathe well throughout the day and during physical and mental work.

Once you have mastered good breathing, we can look at the typical 'calming' disciplines, such as stretching and yoga, how they work, and judge what is best to do. A short guide to 'quick' meditation will help you to clear and focus your mind.

And, although most of us imagine that quiet, meditative exercise as the definitive 'relaxing' exercise, in fact even quite 'active' work enables the body to unwind and calm down, so finally we discuss why you should get moving to help you relax.

The ideal relaxation programme is one that combines all these three areas – breathing, quiet exercise and active work. However, you don't need to spend a great deal of time on all of these, as proved by our 10 Minutes-a-day Unwind. Do it every day and you will quickly find that you have programmed both body and mind to relax almost to order, no matter what stresses each day brings.

breathe ... The way that you breathe is a vital key to relaxation, because it both reflects and controls your body's mental and emotional state.

Few people are even aware of their breathing, or that they are not 'doing it properly' – as, rather like the heart beating, it seems like something that should be completely involuntary and natural.

But not only is our breathing an almost instant reflection of what is happening in our lives, it can also, with practice, control emotions and physical reactions, and thus help to relax both mind and body. No wonder there are numerous sayings involving breath: 'It took my breath away' (faced with an immense surprise); 'I could hardly breathe' (dealing with fear or anxiety). How you feel and how you breathe ... inextricably linked.

When you breathe in, air is drawn into the windpipe and then the lungs via two large tubes (the bronchi) and finally into the network of small airways in the lungs to reach the air sacs. Here the blood vessels absorb oxygen, which is the vital fuel for many body functions – most importantly, the brain and the heart – and which is carried round the body by the blood. Then carbon dioxide is released via the out breath, along with debris such as dust and other unwanted particles.

What is normal breathing? We usually take around 12 breaths per minute, but during physical exercise that can go up to 20 or more, which provides the body with much needed extra oxygen. However, many people have speeded-up breathing, which is shallow, and this is termed hyperventilation. The usual cause of this is emotional stress and/or muscular tension and/or poor posture and, eventually, long-term habit.

Hyperventilation means that the body is not receiving as much oxygen as it should and this can lead to dizziness, faintness, disorientation, palpitations or racing heart, stomach pains, headache, muscular tension, fatigue, anxiety and panic attacks. At times of high stress, the breath may literally be 'held' for periods of time, without the person realizing he or she is doing this, which also causes a lack of oxygen to the brain.

In other words, improper breathing due to stress leads to a vicious circle of more stress and other negative symptoms, which may lead to yet more stress and even poorer breathing.

how do you breathe? You may be surprised to
note you are hyperventilating as you read this. Take a deeper breath IN and then OUT. You get the immediate feeling that you are releasing pent-up tension and your face relaxes a little.

posture exercises to help breathing

Practise standing with good posture Try this against a wall. Stand with your feet 2 inches apart, your knees slightly relaxed, your stomach and bottom tucked in, your ribcage free, your shoulders down and relaxed, your spine straight but with a light curve at the bottom, your head balanced well on your neck, without the chin pointing upwards. Check that your pelvis is in 'neutral' – if it tilts forward your stomach will tend to protrude. Stand like this and concentrate on holding good posture while breathing normally.

chest stretch Stand with good posture as described above. Now clasp your hands behind your back just above the tailbone and bring your arms out behind you as far as you can. Feel a stretch all across your chest. Hold for a count of 10 and return to the starting position. Repeat this several times a day.

check – Lie down and relax with your right hand on your bellybutton and your left hand on your chest. If you see your right hand moving up and down as you breathe more than your left hand, then your breathing (at the moment at least!) is good. More chest movement indicates you have shallow breathing.

AT RISK – People who have stressful jobs which involve a lot of deskwork or driving (both linked to poor posture) and long hours focusing on mental tasks (no focus on the body) are at highest risk of hyperventilation.

relearning breathing Just as poor breathing brings a potentially long list of negative side-effects, so good breathing is an important exercise that can make you feel better, help calm you down, help you to relax in both mind and body. With deeper, regular breathing you will be fully oxygenated with muscles that can relax. Opposite is a 5-step exercise plan for better breathing. Practise it every day in order to overcome your old bad habits.

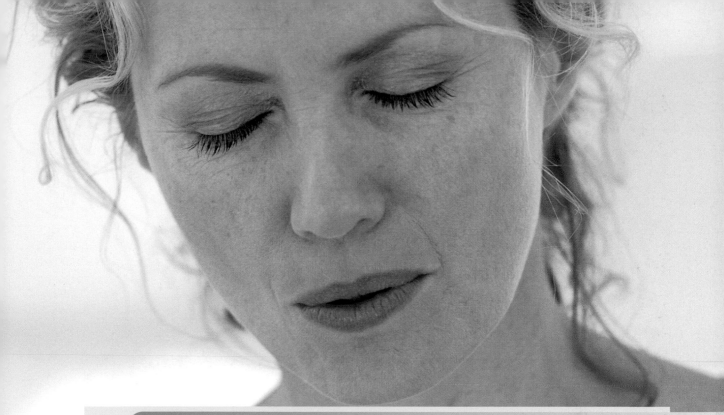

5 steps to better breathing

1 In the morning and in the evening, stand or sit in an upright chair with your shoulders relaxed and back and chest as 'free' as you can manage, hands resting lightly on the lower abdomen.

    Do a 'false yawn' to release jaw tension. Now breathe in through your nose to a count of 5, concentrating on getting the breath down into the stomach area. Breathe slowly out through your mouth to a count of 3–5. (The nose catches pollutants in the air on their way into your body, the mouth allows pollutants to be released from the body.) Do this for 1 minute, using a timer if possible.

2 Aim eventually to get your rate down to 8 breaths a minute. Slower breathing is calming and indicates that you are getting sufficient oxygen into your system.

3 Throughout the day, remember to do this type of breathing in difficult situations and when you feel tense.

4 Find yourself a key so that you remember to keep checking your breathing all day long. The key can be someone or something that appears/happens frequently in your day. For example, it could be your partner or your work colleague, or the 'new message' symbol on your computer, or your cat, or every time you have a drink, or go to the loo. Every time this key happens, it is your reminder to check your breathing.

5 Work on your posture. The correct posture helps to release the chest muscles so that the diaphragm can expand properly, and postural and stretching exercises help release tension in the head, neck, shoulders, back and chest, which also restricts breathing. Do the long body stretch (page 103) daily, the exercises that follow overleaf and add on any of the upper body stretches on pages 75 and 82–3 if you have time. The suggestions featured in the box on posture opposite will also help.

chill ... Slow, gentle, yet deep exercise is a great way to help you relax in both mind and body.

exercise to relax

If you regularly practise stretching (such as in the exercises on pages 75 and 82–3) or do yoga (the positions of these exercises are based on yoga poses) or other disciplines, such as Alexander Technique, Feldenkrais or tai chi, you will soon find that your body is less tense and that you feel more calm and relaxed. Just a few minutes a day are enough to achieve this effect, but longer periods will also help provide other benefits – such as a more toned and supple body, and better whole-body posture. Back pain may also be relieved.

While you do the exercises, don't forget to breathe properly. When holding a stretch or a pose, breathe as described on page 111. Shutting your eyes can often help you focus on the exercise and relax.

1 wall drape

With a small cushion or towel under your lower back, lie on your back with your legs 'up the wall', as shown, knees slightly 'soft' and arms above the head on the floor. Relax into the position and breathe correctly for 1 minute. This pose helps you to release tension, feel less tired and calm down.

Note: For a modified version, use a sturdy dining-type chair and place the lower legs, with knees bent and thighs vertical, fully on the seat of the chair as you lie on the floor.

2 the fish

Lie on your back on a mat, with your legs out straight and arms at your sides, with your upper back supported on a small cushion or folded towel, as shown. Allow your neck and head to stretch down to the floor. Relax into the position and breathe correctly for 30 seconds, building to 1 minute. This pose helps release your chest, helps shoulder flexibility and calms the mind.

Note: For people with neck problems, bring the cushion/ towel up higher to support the neck as well.

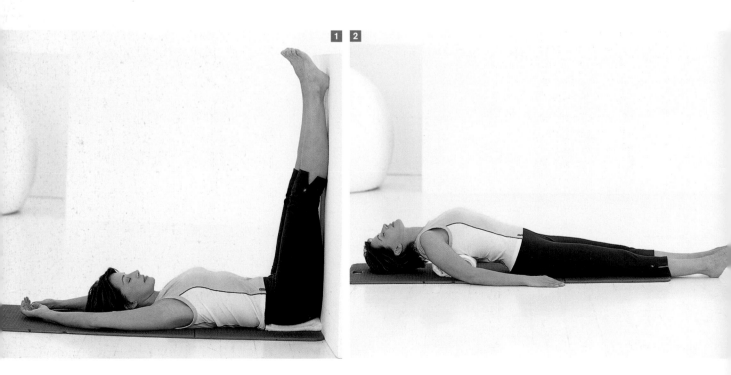

1 2

3 spinal twist

Sit cross-legged on the floor with a small cushion or folded towel under the base of your spine. Breathing correctly, place your right hand on the floor (palm down) near the base of the right side of your spine and turn your upper body and head to look over your right shoulder. Hold the position for 15 seconds, building to 30 seconds, breathing calmly. Slowly return to the starting position and repeat to the other side. This position eases muscle tension in the upper body and frees the chest.

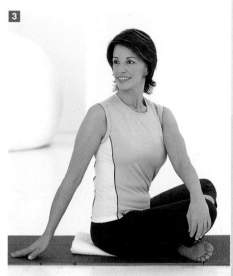

4 cobra

Lie on your stomach on a mat and place the upper body weight on the hands, as shown, looking straight ahead. Hold the position for 30 seconds, building to 1 minute, breathing slowly. This pose stretches the stomach and chest and strengthens the spine.

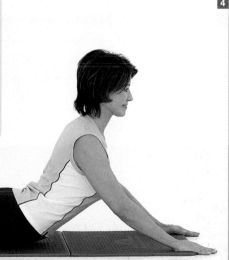

beginning meditation

Meditation can be a good way to relax mind and body, and is an ideal preparation for sleep, especially for people who suffer from insomnia or who have trouble getting off to sleep. There are many forms of meditation, a lot of which require more time and commitment than most of us can give. Here is a simple version.

1 In a warm room, without harsh lighting, and wearing loose, comfortable clothes, sit on a small cushion or folded towel on the floor, either cross-legged (which can be uncomfortable if you are not used to it), or with your back against a wall and your legs outstretched.

2 Close your eyes and breathe correctly into your stomach.

3 When you are ready, slowly say, 'Aaaaah' as you breathe IN.

4 Breathing out slowly, say, 'Huuuuuummmmmm'.

5 Repeat slowly for 2 minutes (approximately).

6 Focus on your body, starting with the head and moving down to the toes, aiming to relax each part of your body as you go, apart from your spine, which needs to stay strong.

7 Sit still and relaxed and try to clear your mind of all stressful incoming thoughts for several minutes, or as long as you need. This is not as easy as it sounds – every time an 'outside' thought comes in, try to replace it by re-focusing on your body and your breathing.

8 Open your eyes and slowly move up.

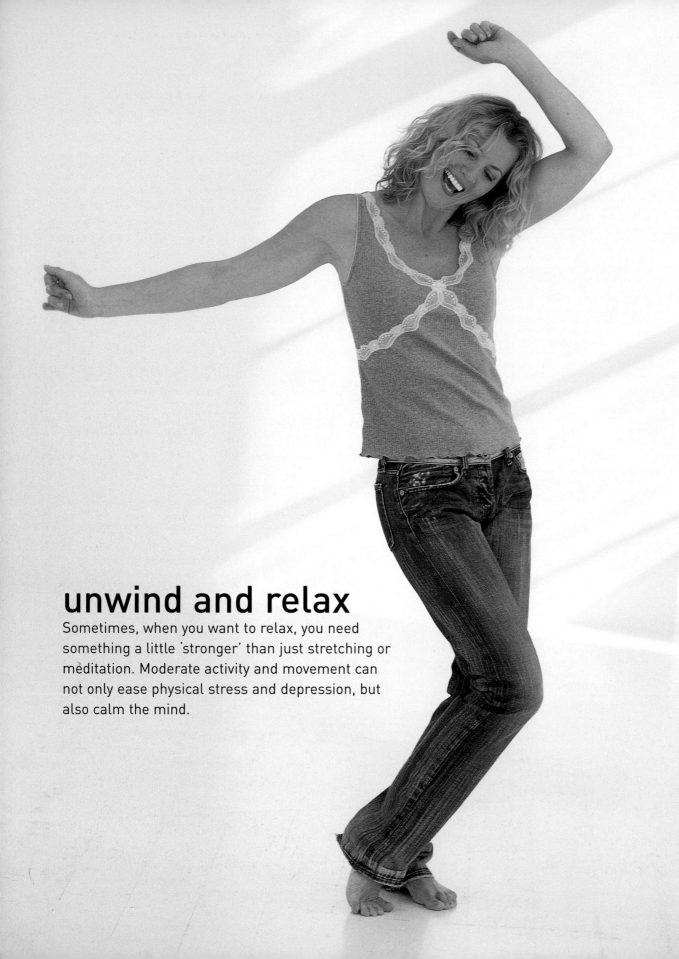

unwind and relax

Sometimes, when you want to relax, you need
something a little 'stronger' than just stretching or
meditation. Moderate activity and movement can
not only ease physical stress and depression, but
also calm the mind.

Why does exercise help you relax?
The main reasons:

hormones at work

When you are physically active, your body releases chemicals known as endorphins. These have been termed 'nature's painkillers' or 'nature's tranquillizers', because they reduce stress and produce a general feeling of well-being. They can also ease depression and lift mood.

Intense exercise, such as hard aerobic work, can release anger and help to clear the mind, while more moderate but long-term exercise, such as a long ramble, can lift depression and improve mood. Research has shown that when people walk for 30 minutes their anxiety levels decrease by 25%. Whether you choose a 10-minute daily walk, 2 minutes' skipping or a 3-hour fast cycle ride, you are helping yourself to feel better.

increased oxygen

While you take any form of aerobic exercise, your lungs are working harder to provide your heart with more oxygen, which is pumped round the body by the blood. This increase of blood and oxygen to the brain helps you to feel better, lifting the mood and, after the exercise, producing an increased sense of relaxation. Some activities which are not aerobic can also achieve increased flow of blood to the brain – e.g. certain forms of yoga.

dispersal of adrenaline

Adrenaline is the hormone released when we are under stress or pressure. It can build up within the body if not dispersed and, experts believe, is linked with an increased risk of heart failure and other stress-related conditions. Exercise helps to rid the body of excess adrenaline and thus helps us relax.

mood manipulation

Certain types of exercise seem to be better for relaxation and mood than others. A crowded session at an aerobics class or an overheated gym might do less to help you relax than all of these:

● Gardening – good for calming the mind.

● Walking in beautiful or stimulating surroundings – good for lifting mood and awakening senses.

● Dancing – research has shown that music is as good as pills for lifting mood (disco-type) or calming (classical or ethnic).

● Sport – a non-competitive sport that you enjoy (e.g. skiing, rollerblading, cycling) does more for your brain than exercise that you find boring.

15 minutes-a-day unwind

Putting together all the ideas in the last 6 pages, here is a sample programme of how you can use exercise to relax mind and body during a typical day:

8.00am
● 1 minute's breathing exercises at open window.
● Chest stretch (page 75) for 1 minute.

8.30am
● 2 minutes' skipping for brain and muscles.

11.00am
● 1 minute's breathing exercises (page 111).
● 5 minutes' walk around your garden or dance to music.

6.00pm
● 3 minutes' meditation.

10.00pm
● 2 minutes' poses 1–4 on pages 112–3. [Chill…]

3

looks for your
newlife

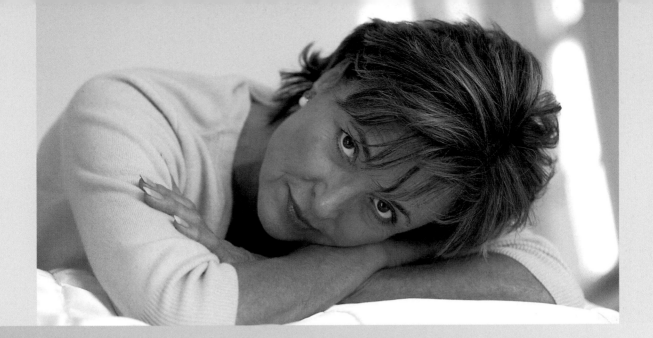

We are all aware that our moods affect the way we look – but the opposite is even more true. If you are looking good, you will feel confident and attractive; if you're having a 'don't look at me' day, you'll feel miserable.

And you can be attractive enough to boost your confidence at any age. In mid life, however, it is not enough just to spend time on yourself – you also need the knack of choosing products, styles and colours that really suit you NOW. You need to avoid the 'too young' or 'too old' traps. You need the courage to let go of the 'old you' and move forward, onward. And you need to keep up to date with the available choices, so all that can be achieved.

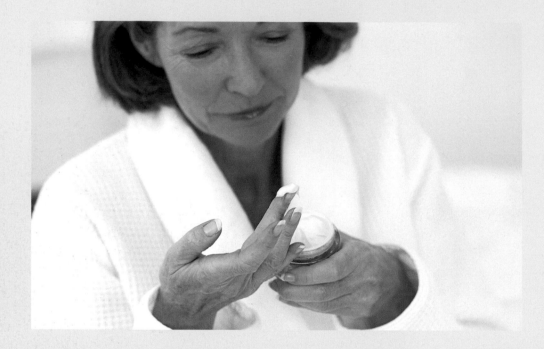

the way we look defines who we are

As we begin to age, however, we seem to take our outer self for granted.

In our 40s and 50s, it is so easy to look in the mirror each day, say, 'This is me,' and proceed to grab the same styles and colours from the wardrobe, put on the same make-up we've been wearing for years and run a comb through the same old cut we've had since 1990. We have, we believe, more important things to think about today.

But, in truth, the way we look remains VERY important. As we begin to age, however, we seem to have fixed ideas on how our outer self should be – if, indeed, we have any ideas at all. Even if we watch our weight and work out to keep in shape, the 'dressing' that coats the body rarely gets a second thought. And when it does, we seem to be led, lemming-like, towards the least suitable item on the fashion rack or the make-up counter. We then get it home, never wear or use it, and don't bother to try again for another year or two.

I believe that we are so used to seeing ourselves that we can't imagine that, over the years, our essential self has changed. We see 'me' in the mirror and, even if there is a small voice shouting loudly 'you need a new look', we tend to ignore it. We have a set of habits – 'our' skin routine, 'our' make-up, 'our' wardrobe, 'our' colours. To change – for change IS, in almost all cases, needed as we age – we need, first, to realize that long-term style solutions no longer work for us and, second, to overcome the natural instinct to hold on to the familiar.

We also need to gauge what is the fine line between looking 'up to date' and looking 'over the top' or – horror of horrors – having any connection with lambs, mutton, dressed as…. We need to achieve a style that is of the time, but still essentially 'us'. And we need to be unafraid to discard what is no longer right for our changing skin and hair texture and colour, and move on. It is rarely best to stick with the same old hairdresser, who has 'known' your hair for 20 years, the same fashion shop, the same brand of make-up you have used since you were 18 and the same skin routine that kicked in at 30.

New may be scary, but when your looks can make such a difference to your life, it is important to try. In Section Three, we help you to bring out the potential and possibilities in your looks – and help you avoid the pitfalls. For whoever didn't – on a particularly bad day – suddenly cry, 'That's it! I'm going to have a facelift and I want it NOW'; or arrive home from a shopping trip with £500 worth of totally unsuitable clothes on a whim. Change and common sense are not necessarily incompatible!

First we look at the secrets of good skin – what makes skin good or bad? What works on your skin at 40, 50 or 60, and what can you realistically expect to achieve at these ages? How to take off 10 years without botox and how to look after your body as well as your face.

Next, make-up… you may need to chuck your old cosmetics to bring your face up to date and make the most of yourself. We give guidelines on trends, products and colours for your age.

If you've ever considered cosmetic surgery, we provide the facts to help you decide, and discuss what could be easier options that can be carried out in your lunch-break. What treatments are really worth the money?

A good haircut can take 10 years off you instantly – we show you how and also discuss colouring and condition. Lastly, we give you tips on repackaging yourself – the clothes shapes, colours and textures that work in mid life for both men and women, and how to wear them. It's a fun ride – so there's no need to worry…

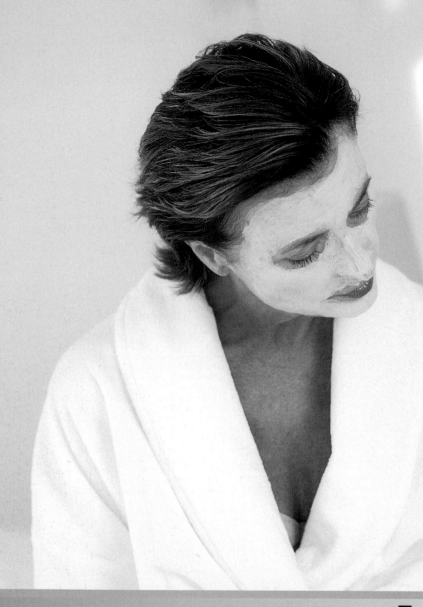

secrets of good skin

While we claim to love our wrinkles for the character they endow and the maturity they represent, we still spend an average of £75 a head each year on skin products ... and many people claim to spend upwards of £50 a week, with the biggest spenders between the ages of 30 and 50. Here we look at what causes skin to age and give all the latest cures and treatments the once-over.

The number-one worry... According to research on facial appearance, the ageing problem that most concerns women is wrinkles. No wonder the face cream market is worth £50 billion a year.

what causes wrinkles? Genetics: your propensity to get wrinkles is to a certain degree mapped out by your parentage. This is the one thing you can't alter, however annoying it is that your best friend never uses face creams and has a peachy complexion with hardly a wrinkle in sight.

sun exposure and pollution Exposure to UVA and UVB rays harms the skin by increasing the production of free radicals (see antioxidants, page 19), which affect DNA, by damaging DNA directly. This damage affects the skin's under layers – the dermis and epidermis – and their ability to produce new collagen (which keeps the skin firm and plump – a lack of collagen means that the skin collapses in on itself and causes wrinkles) and elastin (which keeps it supple). Atmospheric pollution also promotes production of free radicals and thus decreases the skin's self-repairing capability.

Repeated exposure to sun and adverse atmospheric conditions also increases dryness, and skin which lacks moisture is more prone to wrinkling. Some research indicates that if facial skin is 100% protected from the sun from birth, it can still be relatively unlined at the age of 80.

ageing process We all age and there is little we can do about that ... however good your skin and however much you do everything 'right' to keep it youthful, its youthful ability to repair itself and remain fresh, plump, radiant and dewy will diminish over time. Around the menopause, hormonal changes often bring about a sudden seemingly rapid change in the quality of the skin.

There is no cream or lifestyle choice you can make that will keep you looking 18 all through your life, so don't buy any product that promises miracles – but, that said, paying lots of attention to your skin can certainly help slow down its ageing process considerably and help you to look 10–15 years younger.

using your face If you were to spend your whole life not smiling, not frowning and avoiding all facial expression, you would experience many fewer wrinkles on the forehead, around the eyes and around the mouth. However, this isn't a desirable option for most of us, and wrinkles and lines brought about by using our faces are what is known as 'laughter lines' and 'character lines'. They are, in essence, what make you you, and there is certainly plenty to be said for keeping them there and being proud of them. Though, of course, being cheerful and content may lead to attractive, upward looking lines, whereas being bad-tempered and miserable may lead to 'down' lines – not so attractive. A point worth bearing in mind perhaps?

help at hand

If you're still using the same moisturizer or night cream that you did 10 or 20 years ago – ditch it! Cosmetics companies have made huge strides in discovering what causes wrinkles and providing products to help minimize them. While some are hugely expensive, others are reasonably priced and may do as good a job.

Here are some of the wizard ingredients to look out for:

Antioxidants help to prevent free-radical damage. Vitamins C and E are two common antioxidants found in creams, while pycnogenol (pine bark extract) is said to be even stronger. Vitamin C also helps build collagen.

Amino acids These are the 'building blocks' of protein, which is a major skin component and may stimulate skin renewal. The amino acid carnosine has been shown to plump up skin and diminish the appearance of wrinkles; arginine has been impregnated in jeans in Japan to improve the skin condition of wearers, while peptides – another buzzword ingredient – are an amino acid compound which stimulates collagen production, hydrates and firms, and helps to relax the facial muscles, producing a 'botox' effect. These peptides are patented, with names such as Matrixyl and B-neutrox.

Endorphins Hormones that may help to relax the facial muscles and may also produce an effect similar to botox are beginning to appear in several new face creams as I write.

DNA repairers Various marine ingredients seem to help increase DNA repair and slow wrinkle formation – the cosmetic company Lancaster use photolase, an enzyme found in plankton, another plankton enzyme is artemia, while other companies use salmon roe. Actual human DNA components, such as guanine and cytosine, are used in other, expensive creams.

Human epidermal growth factor (EGF) This is another form of protein, released when we are wounded, which helps to speed up the healing process by stimulating cell division.

Plant and yeast extracts Many plants are rich in antioxidants and other skin-repair boosters – green and white tea are now reasonably common cream ingredients while walnut and apple extracts, Japanese pitera (a yeast extract), aloe vera, yucca and sea algae are also favourites.

Retinol (vitamin A) This has been used for several years as a firming ingredient and often appears in cheaper creams.

Alphahydroxy acids (AHAs) These fruit acids may smooth out the appearance of fine lines – but avoid them if you have sensitive skin, as they work via a moderate peeling effect.

Many creams use not just one, but several of these ingredients, which may also help improve other skin problems (see overleaf). Choose a cream after reading the packaging carefully, and, if possible, buy a trial size or get a free sample.

and the other problems …

Dryness Skin tends to become drier as we age, partly because the sebaceous glands below the skin – which produce oil – work less well. For those who used to have oily skin, this can be a blessing. Skin also dries out – i.e. losing water rather than oil – because of wind, cold, sun, other climatic conditions and central heating, and these factors mean it is important to protect the skin with a moisturizer which both encourages oil retention and prevents dehydration.

A cheap moisturizer, containing a mixture of water and oils (such as glycerine, lanolin, paraffin, seed or plant oils), will do the trick, but manufacturers add other ingredients (see above) which may also help wrinkles and other skin problems. EGF (see left), for example, is said to help maintain a 'dewy, moist-looking' skin. Choosing a cream with an added sun protection factor may negate the need for a separate sun block.

Night creams are usually just moisturizer with a lower water content for a thicker product, and tend to have even more 'active' ingredients added than a day moisturizer.

Sagging, thinning skin Sagging and thinning occur due to diminishing collagen and elastin levels (see page 121) and thus some of the creams designed to help wrinkles also help keep skin firm and plump. Creams containing proteins or amino acids typically offer firming and protection from sagging, while vitamin

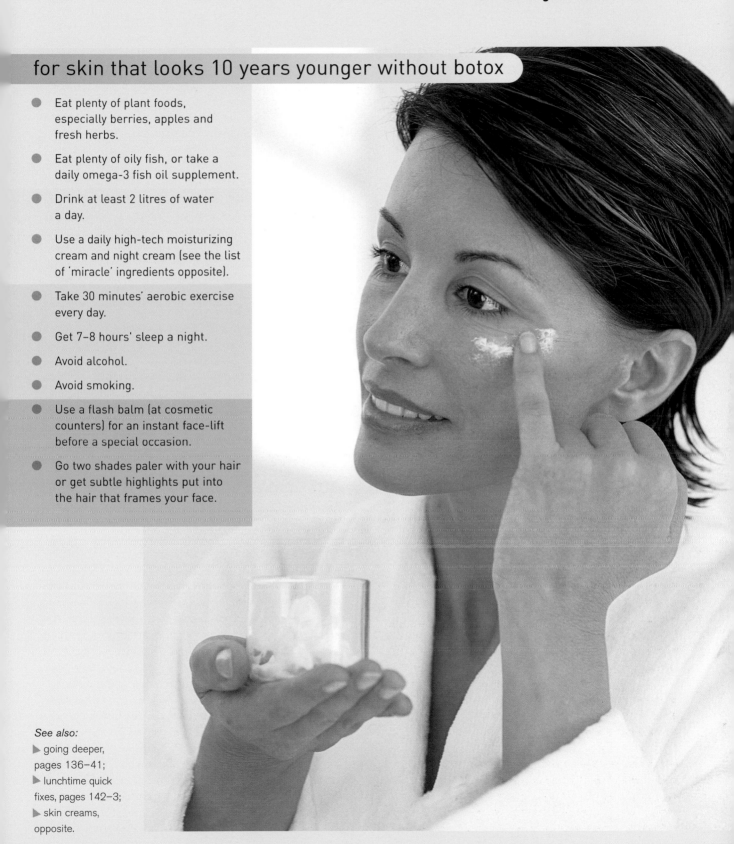

for skin that looks 10 years younger without botox

- Eat plenty of plant foods, especially berries, apples and fresh herbs.

- Eat plenty of oily fish, or take a daily omega-3 fish oil supplement.

- Drink at least 2 litres of water a day.

- Use a daily high-tech moisturizing cream and night cream (see the list of 'miracle' ingredients opposite).

- Take 30 minutes' aerobic exercise every day.

- Get 7–8 hours' sleep a night.

- Avoid alcohol.

- Avoid smoking.

- Use a flash balm (at cosmetic counters) for an instant face-lift before a special occasion.

- Go two shades paler with your hair or get subtle highlights put into the hair that frames your face.

See also:
▶ going deeper, pages 136–41;
▶ lunchtime quick fixes, pages 142–3;
▶ skin creams, opposite.

what to expect at 40, 50, 60
... unless you work at it!

40s Previously oily skin may become drier. Pores on normal or dry skin may look larger due to hormone changes and slower speed of cell renewal. Fine lines are likely around the eyes, mouth, on the forehead and between the brows. Thread veins may appear around the nose and even on the cheeks as the skin begins to thin and the veins are nearer the skin's surface.

50s Skin continues to dry out and needs heavier-duty moisturizing. Wrinkles may appear between nose and mouth, and become more prominent around the lips and eyes. Jawline may be more blurred and a double chin may develop. You may lose fat from your face, making the cheeks look more hollow – a welcome effect for some but not others. Skin is more sensitive and gentler products need to be used. The menopause causes loss of oestrogen, which makes elasticity decline, sometimes quite rapidly.

60s Eyelids may become more heavily wrinkled and crepy, and bags may appear under the eyes (less common in people with good cheekbone structure). Skin is much thinner and paler than 20 years ago, and if exposed to sunlight tends to burn more easily rather than tanning. Use high-protection SPF and fake tan if you like to look golden.

Going on a diet to lose weight around this time may result in deeper facial wrinkles as the layers of fat under the skin disappear and the skin has lost its ability to bounce back.

C may boost collagen production. Sagging also occurs because the underlying muscles are weak and stretched. Dimethyl MEA from Roc and dimethylaminoethanol (DMAE) from NV Perricone claim to have almost instant firming effects by toning the muscles.

Loss of radiance and skin tone Dull skin is a typical sign of ageing, brought about due to cell renewal slowing down. Creams that cause a slight skin peel or dermabrasion, such as AHAs or alpha hydroxy acids (often described as exfoliants or clarifiers) will remove dead cells and make your skin look radiant, but they can be too harsh on older or sensitive skins and, indeed, the US Food and Drug Administration is drafting guidelines for creams containing AHAs to carry a warning that they may increase risk of sun damage. My advice is not to buy these products – look in ingredients lists for AHAs by other names, such as lactic or glycolic acid and sugar cane extract.

Any thorough cleansing programme with a gentle cleanser or soap will help remove dead cells, stimulate circulation to the skin and make you look brighter and younger. EGF (see page 122) also makes the skin look more radiant by stimulating skin cell growth, while a light face massage with almond oil will achieve a similar effect. A weekly moisturizing face mask containing no AHAs will also help improve dull skin.

Thread veins – see Body skin, page 126.

Eye puffiness, bags and dark circles The products most likely to help minimize eye bags and puffiness are special eye gels and masks, or eye contour creams and balms. Gels and masks kept in the fridge may reduce puffiness because they are cooling on the skin, and may contain plant extracts that could have a tightening effect. Creams and balms may help to even out fine lines but will do little to reduce bags and puffiness.

There is little evidence that any cosmetic can remove dark circles under the eyes. Dark circles always look worse if you are tired or stressed, and will also be worse after vigorous or prolonged exercise. They may also be an indication that your cardiovascular system is not as healthy as it could be.

Spots, acne Although acne is often a teenage complaint, many mid-lifers suddenly find they have a recurrence, or get it for the first time in their lives. This is usually due to hormonal changes at menopause, ceasing to use the contraceptive pill, or sometimes to polycystic ovary syndrome, and although a healthy diet (see page 25) may help, you may need to use an over-the-counter cream containing benzoyl peroxide or see your GP for an antibiotic cream or tablets. You should also take care to cleanse your skin thoroughly (see opposite) and get plenty of exercise outdoors. Although sunlight has been shown to improve acne, you need to balance this knowledge with the damage that too much sun can do to your skin in other ways (see above). In time, most mid-life acne caused by disturbed hormones should clear up of its own accord.

Lip problems As we age, lips tend to get thinner, flatter and less firm, and small lines can appear radiating from the lips into the surrounding skin. This can cause lipstick to 'bleed'. There are various creams designed to help improve these problems and, indeed, creams designed to help plump out and firm the skin and ease wrinkles already discussed should also help lip condition. Lip balms and salves can help prevent dryness, chaps and cracks. Several brands of lip primers are intended for use before applying lipstick, and work well to plump lips and prevent lipstick bleed (see Wake up to Make-up, page 130).

Flushing and ruddiness Hot flushes can produce blushing and redness, and the best solution to regular flushes is to spray your face with a cooling water mist from a canister such as Evian (a pocket size is available) and use a fan. A green-tinted foundation can minimize redness.

A ruddy complexion may be the result of a high alcohol intake or a healthy outdoor life, but some people are just genetically prone to ruddiness. Get your doctor to check you over, as ruddiness may have a medical cause.

Cleansing Even if you haven't worn make-up, do a thorough cleanse at night with a gentle cleanser and soft tissues or cotton-wool pads, or with cleanser-impregnated pads (using a separate eye make-up remover wipe if necessary) and then use your night cream or moisturizer. I wouldn't recommend a facial toning liquid, even if you have open pores – it may irritate sensitive skin and research shows that, in fact, such products do nothing to help close open pores that cold water won't do, and the effect is only temporary.

A once-a-week hydrating face mask is also a good idea for most people. With all cleansing products and masks, try not to pull or scrape the skin too much, especially around the eye area.

some more lifestyle tips...

1 Exposure to the sun is a major skin ager. If you keep your face out of the sun and/or use a SPF of at least 15 all the time, and wear sunglasses whenever you need to be out in summer, you should get many fewer and/or deeper wrinkles.
2 A diet rich in essential fatty acids (see pages18–19) can help prevent skin dryness, as can drinking plenty of water.
3 Get enough – but not too much –– sleep. Long hours in bed can make eyes puff up.

facial exercises

Do these exercises twice a day to see real results.

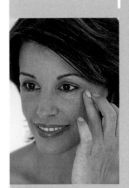

1 To reduce puffiness around the eyes: Use the ring finger of your right hand to do your right eye, left hand to do your left eye. Close your eyes and gently press a finger into the inner corner of your lower eyelid for a few seconds, then move a few millimetres across towards the outer eye, pressing gently again. Continue like this until you reach the outer corner. Repeat with the other eye.

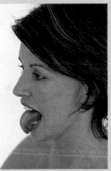

2 To reduce a double chin/turkey neck: Sit with your shoulders relaxed and neck stretched out comfortably long. Now stick out your tongue as far as it will go, until you feel a strong pull across your lower jaw. If you look in a mirror you will see that the flesh under your chin has largely disappeared. This is because the muscles that support it are working to pull it in. Relax and repeat 10 times, trying to hold the tongue out each time for at least 10 seconds.

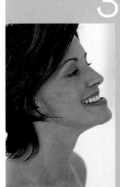

3 Sit with your face and jaw relaxed and look straight ahead. Tilt your head back a little and jut your lower jaw out slightly. Now smile as widely as you can – this will feel peculiar because it is hard to smile while your lower jaw is taut. Clench the back teeth as you do this. Lastly, move the lower jaw up and down slowly 10 times as you maintain the tilted smiling position.

body skin
Even if you are well toned and not overweight, the skin on your body, hands and feet can let you down. Here we look at some of the most common skin troubles in mid life and examine the possible solutions.

dry or wrinkled skin

Body skin can become very dehydrated over time, through sun exposure and the detergents in bath and shower products. There are many moisturizing lotions and creams designed especially for the body which often contain similar ingredients to the face creams but may be richer in oils. There are also products designed especially for the neck and décolletage area, for the feet and, obviously, for the hands. The key to the success of these is regular generous use, rather than expense.

I would say that you don't need a whole array of different creams for different areas – one good rich lotion for large body areas (legs, arms) and one cream for smaller areas with drier or harder skin (feet, elbows, knees) would be sufficient. Also choose cleansing bath and shower products that are as rich in moisturizers and low in chemicals as you can.

For hard-skin areas, you can choose a cream that contains AHAs (see page 122), which have a peeling effect, but avoid using these on more fragile skin. For skin that tends towards eczema and redness, try aloe vera cream or emu oil and see also diet advice for skin on page 25. For skin that looks dull and flaky, you can purchase a variety of body scrubs, smoothers and exfoliators – but I would avoid these if you have sensitive skin (including eczema and redness), as many contain items such as salt, Epsom salts or AHAs.

hands and age spots

Age – or liver – spots on the hands are an easy giveaway of age. It is thought they are caused by free-radical damage and made worse by prolonged sun exposure – but there are some treatments that do seem to diminish the pigmentation. Over the counter you can buy creams containing lactic and glycolic acids and other AHAs (see page 122), which may help by peeling off the outer skin layers and encouraging regrowth. Some creams include high 'doses' of vitamin C, an antioxidant which may help to lighten age spots in time. Such creams may also help to improve the appearance of older hands – e.g. lessen wrinkling, sagging and thinning – and may claim to make hands look more plump, but there is little scientific evidence. Clinic treatments for liver spots and ageing hands have reported successful results (see Lunchtime Quick Fixes, pages 142–3).

cellulite

When cellulite creams have been tested in clinical conditions, results have on average been poor – any 'active ingredients' rarely manage to penetrate deep enough into the skin to reach the cellulite cells – but regular use of a cream (not necessarily expensive) or essential oil mixed into an almond oil base, combined with body brushing or massage of the area, does smooth the skin and improve the appearance of cellulite, without actually getting rid of it. A few expensive creams contain oxygen, said to eliminate cellulite-causing toxins, but most dermatologists are sceptical of this as the appearance of cellulite is not, in any case, significantly caused by toxins, but rather by fat.

Fluid retention can make cellulite look worse, as research shows that while cellulite IS fat, it contains more proteoglycans (water-attracting molecules) than other body fat. The fluid will fill the cells between the connective tissue and plump them out more. Using a good-quality powerful hand-held electric massager, such as the MiniPro Thumper, will stimulate the lymph glands to reduce fluid retention. Diet and aerobic exercise will help to improve cellulite by creating an energy deficit and thus burning off the fat, although even slim people may have some orange-peel on their thighs. Salon treatments for cellulite are discussed in Lunchtime Quick Fixes on pages 142–3.

thread veins

Tiny red veins close to the skin's surface can appear all over the body, particularly on the face around the nose, cheeks and chin, on the legs and on the cleavage. There is little evidence that any cream can remove them – but a fake tan or cosmetics can disguise them. The only way to deal with them, if they really bother you, is to get treatment with light/laser therapy (see Lunchtime Quick Fixes, pages 142–3) or with clinical sclerotherapy (see Varicose veins).

varicose veins

Another sign of ageing that affects one in three people, varicose veins in the legs are unsightly and can be painful. They can be hereditary or may start during pregnancy or long periods of inactivity, and can be worse if you are overweight and do a lot of standing. The muscles and valves that normally pump blood around the body don't work well and the veins become swollen with blood. Regular exercise and weight maintenance are important to help avoid them, and some experts believe that topical cream, supplements or tincture containing horse chestnut and vitamin K may work by helping to tone the vein walls (see also Fuel for your Body, page 8). However, the main line of attack is clinical treatment, sometimes available on the NHS. This may take the form of surgical, laser or radiowave removal, or sclerotherapy, when the veins are injected with a saline solution that makes the vein walls stick together and closes them off. See your doctor to discuss your options.

warts, moles, tags Warts can often be removed by regular use of an over-the-counter ointment, while if you have large moles that bother you, see your doctor, who will advise you. As moles may be cancerous, it is advisable to check them regularly yourself for changes and see your doctor if you spot alterations in size, shape and colour, or itching or weeping. Skin tags are common in ageing skin and, although not dangerous, can be unsightly and are fairly simply removed with surgery or laser – although you may have to pay.

supplements and functional foods

Some pills and foods are sold as aids to good skin – but do they work?

pills Many supplements contain a range of antioxidant vitamins, usually vitamins A, C and E, which 'mop up' free radicals and thus, in theory, will help to prevent ageing. However, most experts believe that these vitamins are best eaten as part of real food. For example, an orange is high in vitamin C but also contains several other plant chemicals which may contribute to the anti-ageing process. For more on antioxidants and eating for skin health, see Section 1.

Vitamin C may also help repair and maintain collagen, while the mineral zinc, found in some skin supplements, is important for skin repair and growth. The plant chemical pycnogenol, one of the bioflavonoid group of phytochemicals, can also help maintain collagen.

omega oils in supplement form can help maintain skin moisture and condition, while supplements aimed at menopausal women may contain ingredients that help minimize skin problems due to hormonal changes.

foods By now, the US dermatologist NV Perricone's 'Facelift in your Fridge' diet (consisting of three meals a day containing the high omega-3-oil salmon) is famous, and 'nutraceuticals' – foods that double as medicines or cosmetics – are now becoming more common in the supermarkets. The market is worth $9 billion in the US and £1 billion in the UK, so by adding nutrients such as vitamins, minerals and phytochemicals to processed foods, manufacturers are hoping to persuade us to buy more. Currently, few of these foods are aimed specifically at skin rejuvenation or maintenance – with the exception of a collagen drink from Japan called Toki – but L'Oréal and Nestlé are working on beauty foods for launch shortly.

male grooming
If your idea of vanity is splashing on a little cologne after your soap and water shave, maybe it's time to think again ... Time was when most men really considered it sissy to have any kind of grooming routine other than the very, very basics ... but if you still think that way, you're out of date.

Today the cosmetics counters are heaving with products aimed at men, and estimates are that the average male now spends nearly £600 a year on grooming products, with some 'urban professionals' spending ten times that much.

In mid life, in certain respects, men need to pay more attention to their 'beauty' routine than women do. Skin condition is paramount because, unlike women, most men don't – and probably never will – wear much in the way of the cosmetics that women rely so heavily upon and which can help to disguise flaws. Also, men tend to have coarser skin and more skin problems than women, because of the different types of hormones that predominate in males. Shaving brings its own problems, including over-dry or sensitive skin, so know-how in that department is very important.

With care, suitable products and just a few extra minutes a day, every man, at almost any age, can have terrific skin and the well-looked-after glow that only comes from attention to detail. And it doesn't need you to take out a second mortgage…

● Buy trial sizes of all new products, if available, so that, if you don't like it, you won't have wasted lots of money.

● If you are prone to open pores, pore strips (available at the chemist) are a good way to remove them quickly.

● Don't forget your daily antiperspirant/deodorant (used after, of course, your daily morning shower or bath). Although not too environmentally friendly, spray is better for men than a stick as the armpit hair prevents the stick reaching where it needs to be – your skin. It is true that men do tend to per-spire more than women do, and because of the under-arm hair, they tend to get more potent BO.

● Don't neglect your fingernails – cut them regularly, bluntly across the top, leaving only a small amount of white (long nails on men are a turn-off).

● Avoid anything but the neatest goatee or perfectly and regularly trimmed beard. Avoid all beards – and even stubble – if your facial hair is grey, or going grey, as they will make you look much older.

● Shave off those sideburns!

● Regularly check that you have no nose or ear hair (highly unattractive to women, even your wife), and remove it with a mini shaver designed for the job. Also trim eyebrows – as men get older, their eyebrows tend to 'bush', and you want to avoid the Denis Healey effect. Pluck the brows to open out your upper eyelids (or get them done while you are at the hairdresser).

● If your brows and/or eyelashes are very pale or grey, consider getting them tinted at a salon. This doesn't take long, isn't painful and the effect will last for weeks without anyone knowing your secret.

● Avoid excesses of alcohol and avoid smoking if you want good skin. Alcohol can give you a florid complexion with broken veins; smoking and alcohol are both drying.

● Younger mid-life males can use tiny touches of make-up – clear mascara for instance, to thicken and lengthen lashes, or good-quality concealer (used sparingly) to hide under-eye tiredness – for evening use only, though. A florid complexion can be damped with a green-tinted moisturizer.

● Don't forget to clean your teeth regularly with a tooth-whitening paste, and drink lots of water to help prevent stale breath. Floss daily and get three-monthly cleaning and descaling at the dentist.

● Check the section on hair for tips on hair care.

● Instead of using after-shave lotions to smell good (see opposite), choose an eau de toilette and splash it behind your neck/on your body/on your wrists.

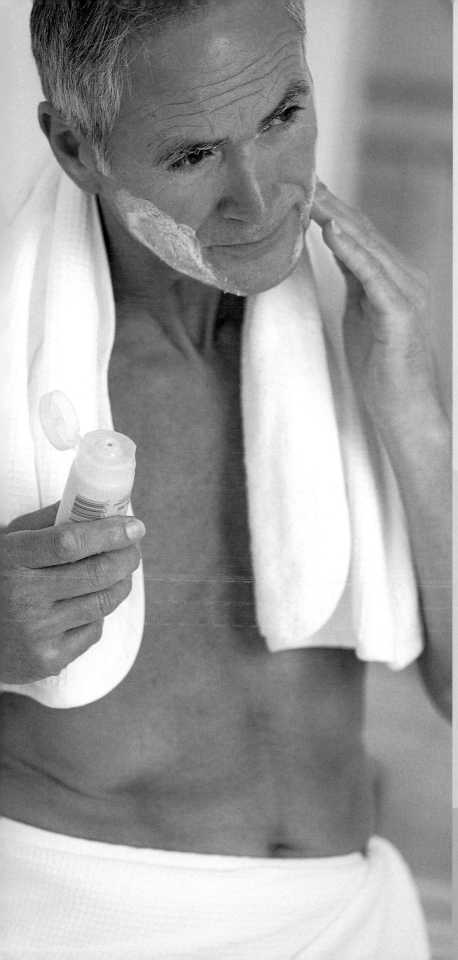

shaving routine

1 cleanse Cleansing with a proper cleansing lotion before you shave not only cleans the skin but also helps to prepare it for shaving. Shaving alone won't cleanse the skin properly, and many brands of soap have too high a pH level, which is acid and drying. If you tend towards oily skin/enlarged pores/blackheads, then choose an oil-free cleanser; if you have dry skin, use a rich moisturizing cleanser. Either way, ensure it contains no alcohol and use cleansing pads to apply.

2 shave Use a rich mousse or gel, not soap (see above). Some contain added moisturizers, which are good even for oily skin. Use a good-quality electric or disposable-blade razor (replace frequently).

3 refresh Splash your face with cold water and/or cleanse off last traces of mousse/gel with a cotton-wool pad soaked in water. Don't use a toning lotion – these don't have any special pore-closing effect and can dry out the skin, especially if they contain alcohol. Shaving removes the top layer of skin (like a peel), which can cause redness and sensitivity, especially as you age, so treat your skin gently after a shave.

4 moisturize Smooth a good unperfumed moisturizing lotion all over face and neck. Choose a very light one if you have oily skin, a slightly richer one for dry skin – choose one that takes no more 30 seconds or so to be absorbed.

5 after shave? Don't use perfumed after-shave lotions! Many contain drying alcohol and additives that sting.

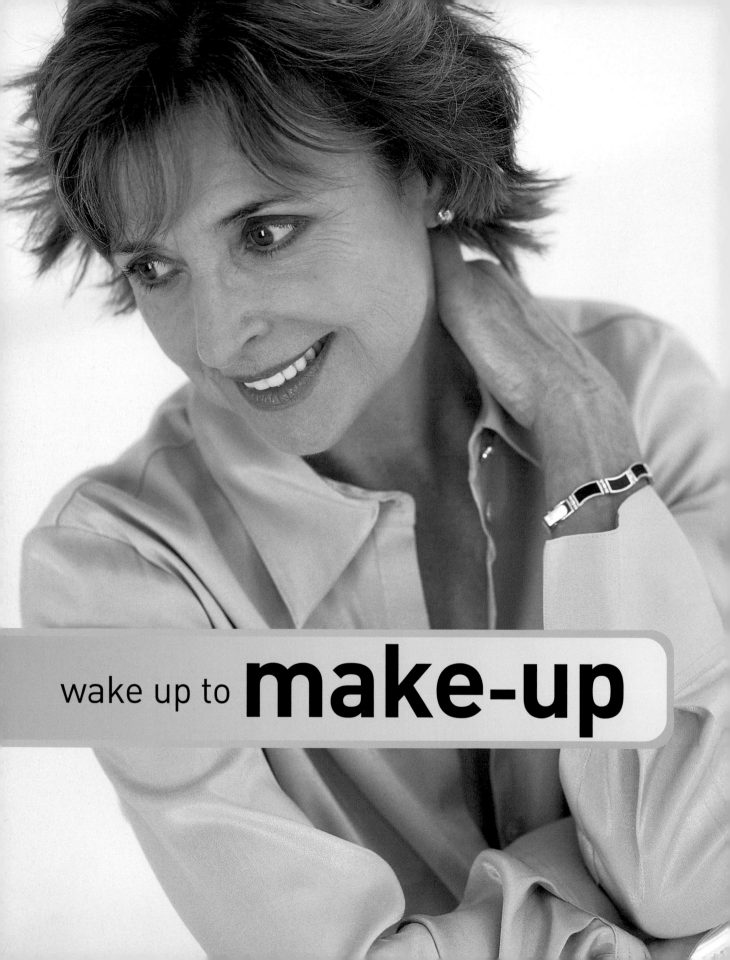

wake up to **make-up**

Make-up, well chosen and carefully applied, can take years off your looks and do a great deal for your confidence. Here we consider the latest advances in make-up and help you decide what is most suitable for you.

Why should I wear make-up? This is a question I have often been asked by women of forty-plus, many of whom feel that cosmetics are for the young, or who believe that wearing make-up gives out the wrong signals.

And yet, if you choose the right products and colours, make-up can help you to look younger, look better and feel more confident. Here are some of the advantages that make-up can achieve for you:

it adds colour As we age, skin colour and tone
become paler. Discreetly applied, items like blusher, lipstick and eyeshadow can return a young bloom to the face.

it adds definition One of the first things you may
notice about your face as you get older is that your features start to lose their definition. Make-up can restore this to thinning brows, brows the natural colour of which is fading, eyelashes that are more sparse than they used to be, and lips whose outline is becoming blurred as the natural rosiness of young lips decreases.

it enhances good points I have seen so many
women of all ages who might be described as plain or non-descript, turn into ravishing beauties after they have put their 'faces' on. For example, if you have pale eyes, brows and lashes, even the most beautiful eyes can be hard to 'see' when people look at your face. The right eye make-up makes them noticeable; a little lipstick can enhance a lovely lip line that may normally be quite pale and hard to notice; and so on.

it disguises bad points If you bring up your
good points with make-up this immediately takes attention away from any less good features … But a little extra care with the cosmetics bag can do some further disguising tricks, especially useful for evening time. For example, thin lips can be made slightly more full with a lip pencil and other new ideas (see page 134). Poor skin texture or uneven skin tone can be disguised with a good foundation; dark under-eye circles can be hidden with concealer; and so on.

it can bring variety and fun into your
life Changing your look with make-up is very easy to
achieve once you have the basics mastered. Using lipstick and eyeshadow (discreetly when it comes to eyes) to tone in with your outfit each day is an easy way to look coordinated and stylish.

it can keep your look up to date As make-up
is relatively inexpensive, it is easy to bring yourself up to date with the latest must-have lip/eye colour or texture.

So don't be shy – let's look in your cosmetics bag and see what we can do …

your cosmetics bag... let's give it a makeover! Here are three simple steps to getting yourself products you'll actually use.

step 1 – do a spring-clean

Take everything out of your make-up bag (and anywhere else that cosmetics may lurk) and sort them through. Throw out ANYTHING over 6 months old which you can't wash. Make-up items such as eyeshadows and pencils, face powders and lipsticks quickly attract a whole range of microbes that can give you infections. One estimate is that 50% of minor eye infections in women are caused by old eye make-up. Old make-up is also likely to be past its best in terms of ease of application. Foundation and nail polish thickens, lipsticks and pencils may dry out, etc. And the colours/textures may be passé.

Wash and thoroughly dry brushes, powder puffs and applicators that are worth keeping. Throw them away if they are worn, old or not fit for the job.

Now throw out anything that is in a colour or texture that you don't like and which you bought on a whim or in error. If you don't like make-up (even if it suits you), you won't feel good wearing it.

Lastly, throw out any foundation, concealer or powder that makes you look over-made-up or caked. As you get older, less really is more, and you need a light touch with a cosmetic that covers your skin.

step 2 – choose your basics

Should you have anything left that fits the bill for any of the following six categories, then you needn't replace that item. Otherwise, go to a good, well-stocked cosmetics counter and choose at least one of each of the following:

Avoid your old brands – it's time for a change – and spend time reading the labels ... cosmetics technology is improving all the time

Foundation The latest foundations give an even coverage without looking unnatural and many also contain conditioners, protection against UVA rays, and anti-ageing ingredients. Look for brands and labels that are specially aimed at women of a similar age and skin type to yourself, and which promise light coverage and a 'light diffusing/light reflecting' effect (or similar words), and then try several colours and brands out on the inside of your wrist. (If you have a tan, you may need to use the top of your hand instead, and buy two – for when the tan fades – rather than one.)

Go for a liquid base that doesn't sink into any wrinkles you may have; products with minimal pigment and a soft sheen rather than a heavy matt look, which can be ageing (although some of the newer skin bases – by MAC, Guerlain, Clarins, YSL – give a matt effect without caking or heaviness).

Avoid heavy bases and very cheap products ... with foundation you usually get what you pay for. Foundation applied over a firming day moisturizer will look even better and will last well – you can even get light-reflecting moisturizers.

If you don't like, or need, a foundation which offers anything but minimal cover, go for a tinted moisturizer or a 'skin illuminator'. Avoid coating foundation with powder – use nothing but the lightest dusting of powder on the nose, if you must.

Eye pencil Choose a soft pencil in a shade which is no more than two shades darker than your hair, if fair or grey. If dark, choose a colour which is up to two shades lighter than your hair. Choose a pencil that can be used for brows and for defining the eyes ... Kohl is too harsh for older eyes. When colouring brows, use a fine, feather touch with a lot of tiny lines to give a natural look.

Eyeshadow palette Choose a palette containing at least four colours and two double-ended applicators. If in doubt, go for more muted colours rather than

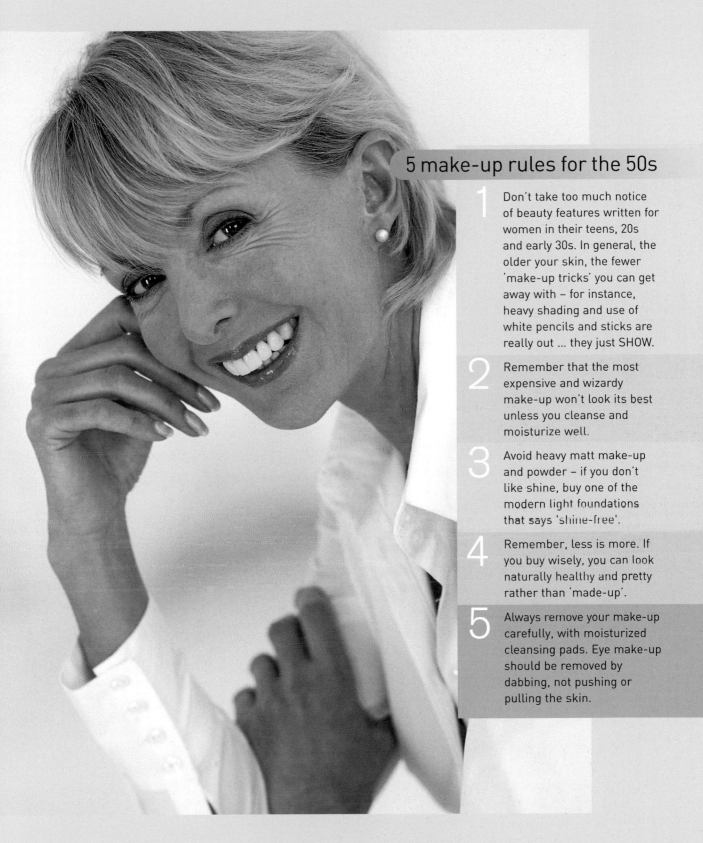

5 make-up rules for the 50s

1 Don't take too much notice of beauty features written for women in their teens, 20s and early 30s. In general, the older your skin, the fewer 'make-up tricks' you can get away with – for instance, heavy shading and use of white pencils and sticks are really out ... they just SHOW.

2 Remember that the most expensive and wizardy make-up won't look its best unless you cleanse and moisturize well.

3 Avoid heavy matt make-up and powder – if you don't like shine, buy one of the modern light foundations that says 'shine-free'.

4 Remember, less is more. If you buy wisely, you can look naturally healthy and pretty rather than 'made-up'.

5 Always remove your make-up carefully, with moisturized cleansing pads. Eye make-up should be removed by dabbing, not pushing or pulling the skin.

brights. Avoid any shiny, frosted or sparkly colours, which accentuate wrinkles, etc. Cream (or, if you have good skin on the eyelids, pressed powder) shadows are best. Avoid anything too dark and blue if you have blue or blue/grey eyes or green if you have green eyes. One colour is usually enough at a time, but if you want to use two (on a large lid area), blend in very well and use colours adjacent on the colour spectrum. Shades of peach, sand, cream and olive complement many older skins.

Mascara Choose a lash-thickening mascara and avoid black. If dark- or olive-skinned, go for brown or dark-grey; if fair and with fair or grey hair, go for mid-brown or mid-grey. Coloured mascaras (e.g. blue, green) are usually a mistake for 40-pluses. Two thin coats are better than one thick one.

Blusher Choose a cream blusher in a shade from your colour spectrum. For most women, peachy-brown and rose-pink colours are more flattering than red or blue-pink. Blusher should be applied, after foundation, with a light hand on the cheek-bones and 'apple' of the cheek, and blended in well.

Lipstick Choose a middle-to-pale shade from your colour spectrum. Dark lipsticks make lips look smaller – an effect you probably don't want, as lips become less full as we age. Straight red and bluey-pinks can be too harsh for older skins and/or grey hair. Lippie with sheen is more flattering than matt, and ensure lip shade tones in well with blusher and eye shades. OR choose a soft blunt lip pencil (a shade at either end is ideal), fill your complete lip in with it and then cover with a thin sheen of gloss.

step 3 – try out and add on

Add to basics what you need for every occasion – ideally 2 eyeshadow palettes (never use both at the same time), 3–4 lipsticks, a lip gloss, a lip pencil in a neutral shade to outline lips before applying lipstick (ENSURE it doesn't show when finished).

make-up tricks

Check here for help with using make-up to best effect for you, and all the top ploys to get the most out of your cosmetics box.

getting clever with make-up

thin lips? Use a lip-plumping base/primer before applying lipstick, to add volume and help to fill in any cracks.

bleeding lipstick? Use a lip fixative/primer to help keep the lipstick in place, or use a lip pencil rather than a waxy lipstick.

eye bags? Use a top-quality concealer such as YSL Touche Eclat UNDERNEATH the bags and use a very light foundation, one shade darker than your other foundation, on the bags themselves.

dull eyes? Go for glossy acrylic-based mascara, e.g. Revlon Lash Lights.

tired eyes? Use peach eyeshadow and blusher.

small eyes? A lash curler will curl the lashes and make your eyes seem much bigger.

double chin? Dust bronzing powder under the chin area with a large soft brush.

dark circles under eyes? Mix concealer half and half with your light foundation and use this, then dust with a highlighter from a compact.

If you aren't sure of your colour type, use sample sizes of make-up, the free testers at make-up counters and small pieces of coloured fabric held up against your face to help you decide what suits your best.

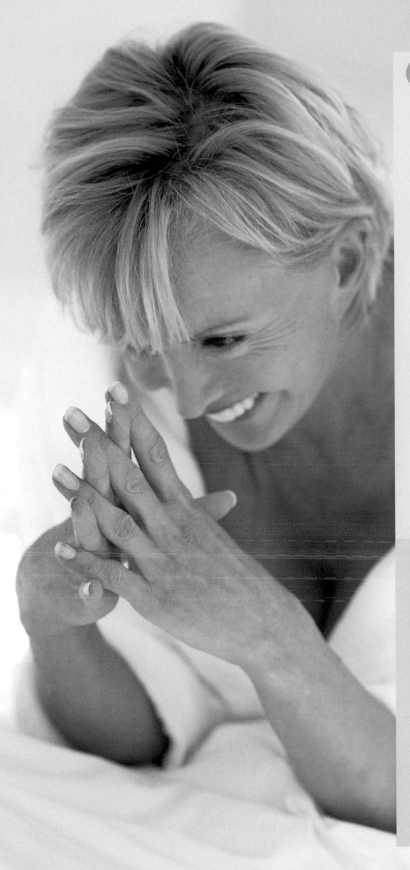

nailing it

Well-manicured nails on both hands and feet show that you care, and they are pleasing and fun.

If you can afford an occasional professional manicure, so much the better - otherwise keep your cuticles in good order by using an old-fashioned orange stick around the nail bases after soaking the nails (in the bath or a bowl of warm water). Invest in a good pair of nail scissors that are really sharp, and cut the nails into a blunt wedge shape rather than the old-fashioned pointy or rounded look.

One marvellous bonus of getting past the 30s is that the older you are, the harder – and easier to grow – your nails become. If they get very brittle, they may chip, though ... so nightly use of a nail-nourishing cream is a good idea. When I remember, I break a vitamin E capsule and rub the lovely oil into the base of my nails, which seems to help.

A French manicure kit will give you lovely white-tipped nails, which always look great and modern. Or go for colour. I never thought I would say this, but you CAN wear blue and green on your nails and it can look brilliant ... but do bear in mind what you will be wearing as, if you aren't matching nail colour to lips – as in the 'olden days' – you need to match it to your clothes unless you are determinedly going for the funky or hippie look. If you are not brave enough for that, a colourless or flesh-coloured polish can make nails look healthy and brilliant.

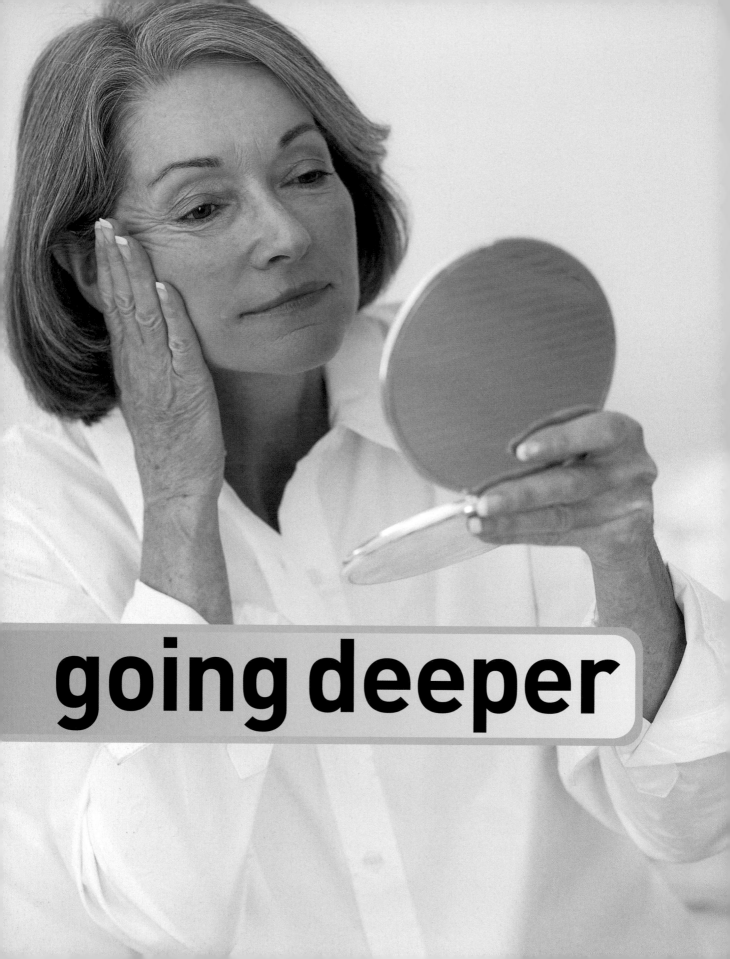

going deeper

Cosmetic surgery, such as facelifts and tummy-tucks, were once the preserve of rich film stars, but now most procedures are almost commonplace, while the range of non-surgical procedures available to everyone is vast.

In the UK, approximately 100,000 men and women now have some form of major cosmetic surgery every year, while – if you include the smaller procedures like blemish removal or skin peels – the figure is nearer 2.5 million. In the USA in 2002, the figure for all (legal) cosmetic procedures was 6.9 million.

Cosmetic treatment is no longer taboo – at least, not for women, although many men are shy about admitting to their facelift or chemical peel. Because it is now so acceptable – even if not yet totally affordable – many of us wonder if this could be the solution to our own physical shortcomings. The cosmetic kings promise a magic cure for every single defect that plagues us from forty-something onwards… eye bags, breast sags, jaw droops, stubborn fat deposits, spare skin, etc., etc. In other words – suddenly, the promise of youthful looks for ever doesn't seem far-fetched any more.

But even the lower-cost operations and treatments are still relatively expensive – many will eat up the cash that might buy you several holidays or a car, while even quickie salon treatment costs mount up if you sign up for a course of ten.

In this chapter we take an unbiased look at what these procedures entail, and whether or not they really are the magic bullet you hope they may be. First we give you the facts on the 'big four' surgical treatments for people in mid life – liposuction, tummy-tucks, facelifts and breast-lifts …. Which variations to choose? Will they work? What are the costs? Who is most suitable for treatment? How long will recovery take?

But before making a decision you need to know the truth about success rates and the dangers, pitfalls and disappointments, so read the Top 20 Things You Should Know.

Lastly, I give you a guide to the popular lunchtime quick fixes – the non-surgical treatments for face, skin, body and shape that take only an hour or so…

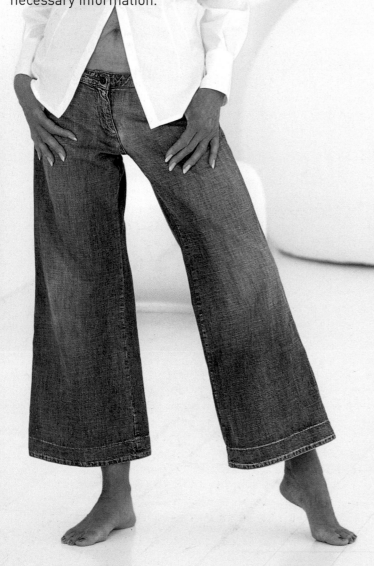

the big four
If you are thinking of having cosmetic surgery, you are likely to be considering one of the 'big four' ... the operations that most interest people over 40. Read our guide for all the necessary information.

liposuction

Liposuction (lipoplasty) is a technique where excess body fat is removed through a tube with a vacuum device. An innovation is the tumescent technique, which is similar, but the fat is pre-treated with a saline solution under local anaesthetic, causing less bruising and swelling. Liposuction is primarily for subcutaneous fat (just below the skin) rather than deep body fat. Another new technique is ultrasound-assisted lipoplasty, which works more efficiently on larger volumes of fat and cellulite.

The best candidates for liposuction are people who are not greatly overweight but have areas of the body where pockets of unwanted fat appears and is hard to shift via normal dieting and exercise – e.g. saddlebags, thigh fat.

Local or general anaesthetic is needed and the effect is permanent – fat can't reappear, because the actual fat cells have been removed. Full recovery takes from one to six months. From £2,000.

tummy-tuck

Also known as abdominoplasty, the tummy-tuck removes sagging/loose skin from the stomach area and is particularly used for people who have been very overweight – in older age, the skin isn't elastic enough to return to normal via exercise. It is also used in women whose skin has been stretched beyond the point of no return through pregnancy.

Excess fat and skin are removed and the muscles of the abdominal wall may be tightened. The effect is permanent – and performed on women only, when they have had their last child. It is rarely done on over-60s and not for people intending to lose a lot of weight (can be done afterwards). Usually done under general anaesthetic. From £4,000.

breast-lift

The breast-lift (mastopexy) raises and reshapes breasts sagging due to pregnancy, weight loss or age, and is most commonly performed on women aged 35-50, preferably who have finished having children (further pregnancies can produce more sagging even after the op). The procedure is carried out by removing excess skin and repositioning the remaining tissue and the nipples. It is often done under general anaesthetic and the results are usually semi-permanent, but not as long-lasting in women with heavy breasts. Leaves noticeable scars, which will be covered by a bra. There may be some permanent loss of feeling in the nipples. Breast implants may be added during the operation to improve the overall bust shape. Cost is around £5,000 plus.

facelifts

Basic facelifts (rhytidectomy) – where the skin was literally hoisted up the face and resewn into position – were the only option fifty years ago. Those having them were considered vain and ridiculous, and results were often not worth the pain and cost.

Nowadays, techniques have improved immensely and there is a choice of several types of facelift to suit most needs. Costs start at around £2,000 and go up to £5,000, depending on type. The panel opposite describes in more detail what happens when you have a full facelift, a brow-lift or a SMAS-lift (lower face). All of these facelifts (plus other options that are available, such as liposuction to remove neck fat during the operation) are major operations, which will be painful and will need several weeks or months of recovery before the face is 'back to normal', and the results should last for up to 10 years. Other popular options are listed below.

Eyes Eyelid surgery (blepharoplasty) removes bags and/or surplus skin on the upper and/or lower lids and corrects drooping, but doesn't remove all wrinkles around the eyes – combined laser surgery can achieve this.
COSTS Around £3,500 for full cyc-lift; £2,500 for eye bag removal. Extra for laser work.
SIDE EFFECT Discomfort, tightening, swelling, bruising, dryness or tearing, sensitivity to light, temporary blurring or double vision.
RECOVERY Able to read after 2–3 days; back to work 7–10 days; bruising and swelling gone in several weeks.
EFFECTS Permanent or virtually so.

Facial implants Implants can change the basic shape of the face, improving a weak chin, poor jaw-line or cheekbone structure, for example. The effects are usually permanent as the implants don't degenerate over time. Cost around £1,500–£3,000.

which facelift?

Traditional facelift: The original one where the skin only is pulled up the face over the muscle and fat, and repositioned. Most suitable for older people wanting younger-looking cheeks and neck. The one that is perhaps most easy to spot. About £4,000

SMAS-lift: The most popular facelift in the UK, this also repositions the facial fat and muscles for longer-term results, including neck improvement. It is especially good for wrinkle reduction, skin smoothing and tightening up the jaw. It should achieve a natural-looking result. However, the skin needs to have some elasticity remaining, so is most suitable for people in their 40s and 50s, or perhaps early 60s. About £5,000. Extended SMAS is also available (most popular facelift in the USA), which has more effect around the nose and mouth and on vertical lines there.

Browlift: Lifts the muscles and skin of the forehead to eliminate sagging, lifts the brows and thus improves the look of the eyes, and minimizes browlines and furrows. Costs £2,000 plus. Another type of upper facelift is the endoscopic facelift, which includes the cheeks, costing from £5,000.

Both these lifts are best for people who still have a good jaw- and neck-line.

Lip enhancement Lips, which tend to thin out as we age, can be improved on a semi-permanent basis (unlike collagen injections – see Lunchtime Quick Fixes, pages 142–3) by using fat (often your own body fat, which has less chance of allergic reaction), GoreTex (a man-made alternative to collagen) or Alloderm (see overleaf), or they can be reshaped to appear plumper with surgery. Both treatments need local anaesthetic. Cost £500 plus.

Facial resurfacing Dermabrasion skims the top layers off the skin mechanically; laser treatment has a similar effect with a laser device; chemical peeling with phenol or other acid removes skin by chemical action. Each helps improve scars and wrinkles, and to even out pigment by encouraging new skin to form. Needs local anaesthetic and produces acute sun sensitivity; 2 weeks off work, and skin redness may persist for months. Prices vary from about £2,000, and more than one treatment may be necessary.

top 20 things you should know...

Before you go ahead with a cosmetic surgery operation, you need to know as much as possible about maximizing the chances of a successful op, and about the cons as well as the pros.

1 Successful surgery depends on the skill of the surgeon. Apply to your country's official plastic surgery association for a list of qualified surgeons in your area. In the UK this is the British Association of Aesthetic Plastic Surgeons, in the USA it is the American Society of Plastic Surgeons, for instance. Their web sites also provide unbiased pros and cons of various cosmetic ops. Your GP should also be able to refer you to someone reputable.

2 Try to find out how much experience your potential surgeon has in the field you are interested in and ask to see his CV and 'before and after' photos.

3 In the UK, a nationwide survey has revealed that some clinics fail to make checks on the qualifications of practitioners they employ.

4 The same survey found that it was fairly common for misleading statements to be made in the advertising of cosmetic surgery.

5 A UK *Health Which?* survey of twenty-one clinics found that people were recommended surgery when they did not need it, and risks were played down or ignored.

6 Make sure you meet the surgeon who will be doing the operation and not just a 'salesperson' or counsellor. Remember, counsellors are not qualified to talk to you about the medical aspects of your intended surgery, or whether it is right for you.

7 A high percentage of cosmetic surgery is done under local anaesthetic, where you will be given a sedative and then anaesthetic – via injection only – around the area to be operated on. If you are squeamish you may not like this. However, general anaesthetic (which renders you unconscious) carries more risks.

8 After cosmetic surgery, skin tends to continue ageing as normal, so even though the effects of the operation itself may be permanent, you may however need another operation in the years to come.

9 Because the word 'cosmetic' comes before the word 'surgery', that doesn't mean your chosen operation isn't serious. Full facelifts, breast-lifts, tummy-tucks, some liposuction, for instance – all are major operations, with the resultant risks and recovery time.

10 Commonplace side-effects of surgery include numbness in and around the site of the operation, bruising, swelling and pain.

11 The ideal age for a first facelift is between 45 and 55. At this age, you still heal fairly readily and if you leave it too late in life the results are usually not so good.

12 Permanent lip enhancement may be carried out using alloderm – made from skin from human corpses, which is washed, freeze-dried and then reconstituted with saline solution before being implanted in the lips. Before having any form of implantation cosmetic surgery, make sure you know what materials are being used, and that you are happy with them.

13 Scarring from cosmetic operations is often played down, but, depending on your skin type and other factors, it can be permanently visible, and scars may be red, uneven and raised. Poor healing and wider scars are common in smokers.

14 More people are going abroad and having cosmetic surgery while on holiday. South Africa is a popular cosmo-holiday destination. Prices are up to 50% lower than in the UK, but the standard is as good.

15 Complications of cosmetic surgery include infection, bleeding, blood clots, adverse reactions to anaesthesia and prolonged tiredness. Individual types of operation carry their own risks: e.g. breast-lift – permanent loss of feeling in the nipples; chemical skin peeling – skin allergies, cold sores; eyelid surgery – difficulty in closing eyes, blindness; facelift – nerve injury; implants – hardening of tissue around the implant.

16 In Florida, USA, a patient died after being injected with industrial-grade silicone which leaked into her bloodstream. The surgeon was charged with third-degree murder. This silicone is often used by unscrupulous doctors in the USA as it is cheaper than safer fillers such as Restylane or Nu-fill.

17 For men who have facelifts, there is a permanent need to shave behind the ears, where beard-growing skin has been repositioned.

18 After dermabrasion or chemical skin peeling, patients need to stay out of the sun for around six months.

19 Liposuction is potentially one of the worse operations for possible unwanted side-effects. The risks include asymmetry (e.g. if saddlebags are done, the result may be uneven to either side); rippling or skin bagginess where fat has been removed; toxic shock; infection and – with UAL (ultrasound version) – thermal burn injuries.

20 Cosmetic surgery may make you look better, but is unlikely to be the complete magic bullet for making your life better. And there is never a 100% guarantee that the job will turn out as you expected it to.

lunchtime quick fixes

Instead of using your lunch hour to go shopping or have something to eat with friends, you could go along to one of the many clinics or salons specializing in quick-fix cosmetic procedures that seem to offer many of the benefits of surgery without the time, pain and cost involved. We look at some of the options from top to toe.

face fixes

wrinkles
You can be injected with various fillers to plump out facial wrinkles. The original collagen (a moisture-retaining protein obtained from animal cartilage) works well on lips and mouth, less well on brows, and lasts 3–4 months. About 3% of people are allergic to collagen.

Alternative fillers are restylane/perlane (hyaluronic acid), a thicker, synthetic gel and a less allergenic filler than collagen; good for crows' feet and nose-to-mouth lines; effects lasting 6–12 months. In some countries you can also get alloderm and silicone (not used so much these days because of side-effects);. £200–400 for a session.

fine wrinkles
can also be softened with IPL (see Veins and marks).

Botox is currently the trendy way to remove frown lines, crows' feet and between-eye furrows. You are injected with botulinum toxin, a bacterium which paralyses the muscles that cause lines. Results are noticeable in 3–10 days and the effect lasts 3–6 months; treatment costs around £250–300 a session. New research indicates that up to 44% of users suffer side-effects, including drooping brows/eyelids, nausea and headaches.

Electrical acupuncture (ERP) is claimed to treat wrinkles as well as open pores and broken veins, but the scientific research on its efficacy is minimal.

veins and marks
Veins on the face, blotchy skin and other marks can be treated with Intense Pulsed Light (IPL) – sometimes called photorejuvenation. Different wavelengths of light (unlike laser, which has only one wavelength) reach different layers of the skin and can treat thread veins without a great deal of soreness or long-lasting redness. Also good for acne scars, age spots and sun damage – even tattoo removal. Several sessions usually needed; from £200 each.

IPL is now preferred to sclerotherapy as the treatment for thread veins (where they are injected with a saline solution), although the latter is less expensive and can also be carried out in short sessions at around £150 a treatment.

skin conditioning treatments High-tech or new age 'superfacials' (sometimes called natural facelifts) can make you look younger by improving the condition of the skin, relaxing or firming the muscles, refining pores, improving lymphatic drainage and so on.

Treatments may consist of a facial massage by hand or machine with essential oils, cream that may contain ingredients such as aloe vera, seaweed, pitera, antioxidants, and/or masks (paraffin wax/plant extract/collagen creams), and/or treatment by hot stones, acupressure , ERP (see Fine wrinkles), electrotherapy, vacuum, steam or brushes – to name a few. The choice is vast and costs range from about £25 up to £75 a session.

Dull, rough or ageing skin, fine lines and pigments can also be treated in the lunch hour with light peels, which remove the surface but aren't as invasive as deep laser or chemical peels. These light peels are often based on fruit acids or salt crystals, sometimes with pressurized oxygen therapy and a finishing moisture mask. It is sometimes claimed that these light peels also stimulate collagen production and may be called microdermabrasion. Prices range from £65 to £100 per session.

mouth: Thin or wrinkled lips can be injected with fillers (see Wrinkles). The outline can be enhanced with semi-permanent lip liner treatment (about £400) or you can have a complete lip blush (filling in the line as well) for around £800. N-Lite laser treatment removes fine lines around the lips from £80 a session (several treatments needed).

teeth can be whitened semi-permanently in an hour, using a mixture of hydrogen peroxide or chlorine dioxide (bleach) plus intense light treatment. Costs £450–750, but not suitable if you have veneers or other synthetics in your mouth.

neck, cleavage and bust

neck Neck-'lifts' are offered, usually based on similar principles to the salt crystal/oxygen treatment for the face (see Skin conditioning treatments). Cleavage treatment can also be included. From £60. A sagging neckline can be treated with electrical impulses to tone the muscles, but the effects are temporary unless treatments are regular. From £40.

Botox (see Fine wrinkles) can be injected to remove wrinkles from the neck and cleavage temporarily, while collagen can be injected into the neck and cleavage for a slightly longer-lasting effect.

A sagging bust can, it is claimed, be lifted by a CACI contour treatment using electrical impulses to firm the pectoral muscles; £25 for 30 minutes (10 sessions recommended).

body

stretchmarks from pregnancy or having lost weight can be improved with laser treatment combined with electric microcurrent and ultrasound.

cellulite There are several different types of salon treatment claiming to cure cellulite, but only endermologie – using handheld massage rollers and suction over a fine mesh suit, which you wear – has been shown actually to work. From £40 for 35 minutes. Users also report good results with ionithermie (clay mask followed by electrical current) and pressurized oxygen treatment, although these haven't been scientifically evaluated to my knowledge.

inch loss 'Slimming' treatments generally rely on some form of body mask (which may contain one or more of a range of ingredients – e.g. vitamin C, co-enzyme Q10, collagen, aloe vera, seaweed, algae, caffeine) topped with a wrap (bandages, cling film). There may also be manual or electrical massage to encourage lymphatic drainage via increased urine output, radio waves or oxygen jet sprays. Experts say that no fat loss is possible through these treatments, only loss of fluid, which will return within a day or two of treatment. Useful for emergency treatment to fit in a tight dress, for instance. About £25–40 for a treatment.

hands and legs

hands Ageing, rough hands can be treated with salt or fruit acid peels (see Skin conditioning treatments) or laser, which does cause the skin to turn red and form a scab, but is better for removing age spots.
Hot wax treatment can smooth and firm the skin, while oxygen booster treatment can plump up and firm the skin. For longer-lasting plumping, restylane (see Wrinkles) can be injected. Costs from £100 to £500.

legs Thread veins on legs can easily be treated with sclerotherapy or with IPL (see Veins and marks).

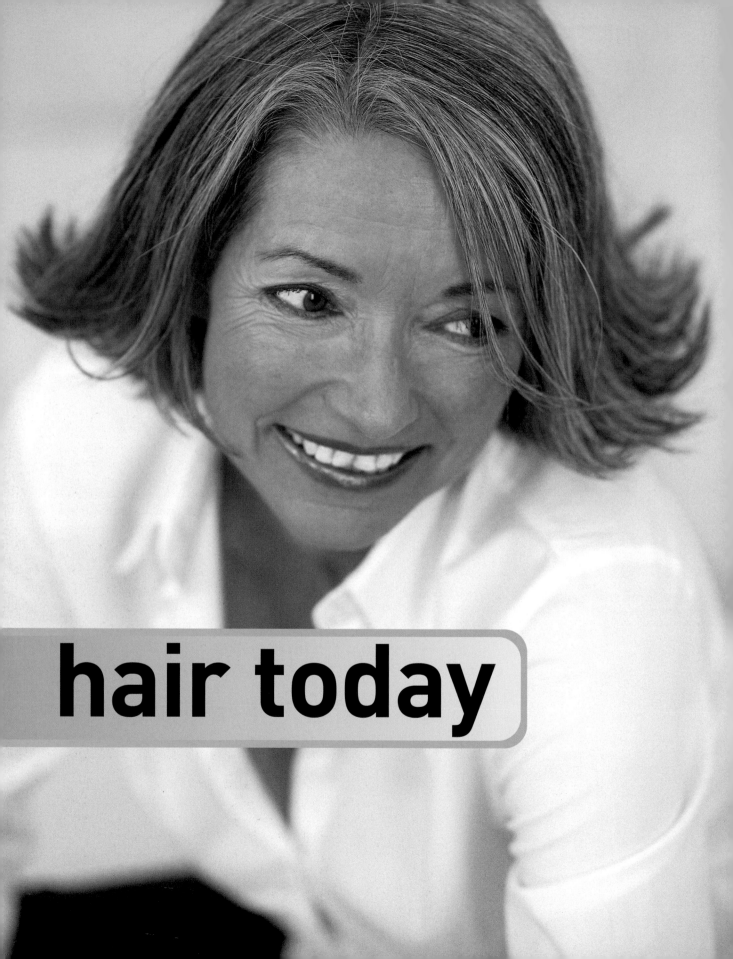

hair today

Research indicates that it is hair that makes the first impression, so no wonder that seven women out of ten worry more about their hair than anything else about themselves except their weight. In mid life things can start to go wrong ... here's how to have the best hair of your life. Clothes, make-up, hair – which do people notice first when they see someone?

If your hair looks good, you will feel terrific, because everyone knows that the right style and colour can literally transform you. A style can take ten years off your age, re-balance your face, hide faults and accentuate your best features, as well as spelling out how you want others to see you – sophisticated, relaxed or glamorous, for instance. And a good colour or colours can also take off years, make you look healthier and enhance your natural colouring.

Because of these obvious advantages of a good hairstyle and colour, it is surprising that many of us, despite all those pounds spent on trying, don't make as much of our hair in mid life as we should. It could be that we get bogged down with the negative effects of ageing on our hair.

It is also true that as we age hair may need more love and attention than it did in youth. For some people, hair goes grey or loses its natural colour, becoming nondescript. It may also coarsen, become more limp or start to thin. Some of these changes can be related to the menopause (or, in males, loss of testosterone), while in younger women hair problems tend to be worse in the premenstrual days. Good nutrition can improve hair condition, while stress and illness can have negative effects.

However, the good news is that whatever your hair problem there is always a solution. Today we have a range of cleansing, conditioning and styling products that will solve any problem, along with fantastic colourants, hardware that has come on in strides in the past ten years, and a wide choice of excellent, well-qualified hairdressers all across the country. There's no need to settle for hair that is anything less than great in mid life, as the pages ahead prove.

fixing solutions
What's your hair problem? Whatever it is – you'll find the answers on the next few pages.

As you get older, you tend to need different products and regimes for your hair. What worked a few years ago may not work for you now,. Spend an hour or so in the chemist's, reading all the labels, and choose products that most closely match your own hair problems (see Styling products, page 151). If necessary, have one set of products for 'normal' days, and another for the times when your hair refuses to behave, e.g. just before a period.

You also need to ensure that you have the best haircut you can get – even the best of hair won't behave if you have a poor cut. Discuss your styling problems with the best hairdresser you can afford to visit and give his or her solutions a try.

'I want a style that makes me look younger'
The quickest way to younger looks is to go for a shorter cut – anything below shoulder level will add years to most faces, and anything below jaw level also doesn't work for many older women. If you really can't face cutting off longer hair, then consider putting it up most of the time – 'up' hair takes years off you too, but leave some fronds around the face, otherwise the look may be too severe. By the way, if you pull hair back off the face firmly it can give you an instant facelift by pulling back the skin!

Unless you have very fine or thin hair, it also helps if the style is 'cut into' – creating tapering or uneven layers and thinning it out. Hair feathered around the neck and ears is also a good look.

Solid block styles all one length are ageing, especially if your hair is heavy, when it 'pulls your face down' by creating more volume at the bottom than the top. Over-'set' hair spells granny if you're 40 plus (even when beehives and set hair are temporarily in fashion), so avoid any hairdresser who wants to give you anything that feels solid to the touch, is coated with spray or doesn't have some movement.

A choppy fringe is also a young look and can help to disguise wrinkles round the eyes and forehead. Avoid a centre parting with no fringe, as this makes the face look longer and older. By the way, if you are dark, going two shades blonder or having highlights makes you look younger too.

'I'm bored with my hairstyle'
Change your hairdresser. The stylist you have used for years will be taking you and your looks and hair for granted, and it can be hard for that person to see you afresh. Take along a few cuttings from magazines to show your new stylist some looks you like, and follow their advice.

To save too much of a shock, change in two stages. For example, from long to shorter on the first visit, then shorter still on the next. If you basically like your style, you may find that a change of colour will be all you need (see Colorants, page 151).

'help – I'm going grey'
Although people generally don't like it when they see the first grey hairs, which seem to shout 'You're getting old!', in fact grey – like blonde – can be very flattering for older skin tones.

If you don't like it, though, rather than try to deal with it yourself I would recommend getting advice from a good colourist, as the best solution varies depending on the amount of grey, your skin, etc.

If you decide to go with the grey, keep it well conditioned, as it can often appear dull. Some people also find that, as they grey, their hair tends to thin out too (see 'My hair is thin and limp' page 148). Experts say grey hair is rarely coarse, but most women find odd stray coarse grey hairs do appear. One or two can be pulled out (don't tell the trichologist!), but for generally coarse hair, a weekly deep conditioner and tongs or a straightener should help.

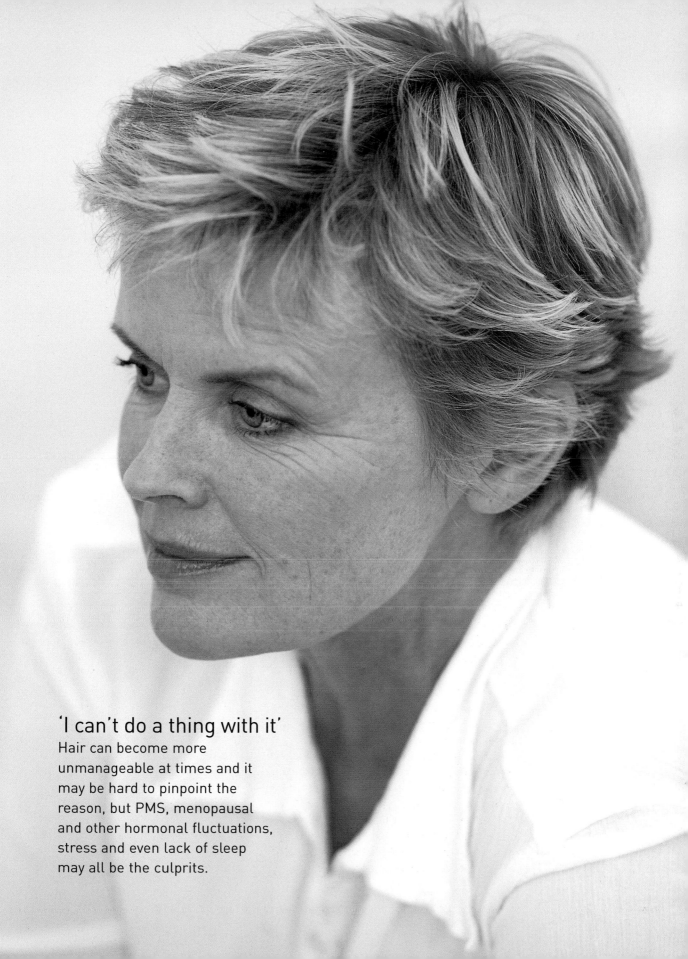

'I can't do a thing with it'

Hair can become more unmanageable at times and it may be hard to pinpoint the reason, but PMS, menopausal and other hormonal fluctuations, stress and even lack of sleep may all be the culprits.

'my hair is dry and frizzy'

Hair does tend to dry out as we age because the body's natural levels of oil production from the sebum glands reduces (why we also get drier skin). Colouring and bleaching can also make hair lose its shine. The answer is to change your products from those you may have been faithful to for years to those with more moisturizing and smoothing potential (see Styling products, page 151). Also use a weekly moisturising mask or hot oil treatment.

Make sure you are drying your hair thoroughly when you style it. For frizzy hair, tongs and straighteners usually smooth the hair out better than drier and brush, which tend to make it more flyaway. Use styling products, like blow-dry lotion, leave-in conditioner, mousse or whichever suits you best.

'my hair is thin and limp'

Just when you want short hair, you find your hair is becoming thinner and more floppy. Greying hair is prone to looking thinner, as the white hairs which produce the grey are finer than your original hair. In fact, over time everybody's hair does thin, because the hair follicles shrink and therefore produce hairs with a smaller circumference. If you started out with fairly thin hair, the problem will be more obvious as you age. The actual number of hairs on your head will also reduce as you get older, contributing to the thinning effect. This is because the ageing process tends to make the follicles lose flexibility and their ability to produce new hair literally dies. This effect is more pronounced in some people, partly due to genetics, but it may be staved off by good diet and regular exercise to increase blood supply to the scalp.

There is evidence that the contraceptive pill and HRT can cause hair-thinning, but not all brands may do this. If you suspect this may be the case, consider swapping to another brand. Thyroid problems may also cause the hair to fall out, so get your doctor to do a thyroid test for you. Lastly, some anti-inflammatory drugs can cause hair thinning if used regularly.

There are plenty of products that help give hair a thicker look, so swap to these, and to help prevent flopping and limpness, use gel or wax specifically designed to retain your style (see Styling products, page 151). Also, use a lightweight conditioner concentrated on the ends rather than the roots. Heavier creams make the hair flop with the extra weight.

for men

Whatever your hair type, you can improve your looks considerably with some know-how and time.

the bald question

Although up to 10% of women have some degree of hair thinning in mid life, baldness is predominantly a male problem, affecting about 70% of men over 40 to some degree. In recent years, the 'trendy' solution has been to simply give the hair a 'number-one' cut all over or even to shave it off completely. This can be a perfect solution, especially if you have a good head shape and the confidence to carry it off. But if that is not your ideal – what can you do?

In recent years, drug companies have developed treatments which are said to stimulate hair growth, but not everyone achieves good results with them. As they are not expensive, however, you could give them a try. In the UK, Regaine is the leading brand name to look for. Alternatively you could try the Advanced Hair Studio's hair replacement system, which, it is claimed, is the nearest you can get to real hair without surgery. Lastly, there is transplant surgery, which is quite expensive and time-consuming, but should last you a lifetime. The Institute of Trichologists can help with more information and details of surgeons. Either way, it is believed that a real cure for baldness is on its way and could be with us within twenty years or so.

Whichever option you choose – please do avoid a Bobby Charlton. The low-parting, combed-over look has become a national joke – don't let the joke be on you. Many men who have found the courage to abandon such a look – possibly even shaving their heads – have been amazed to find themselves looking decades younger.

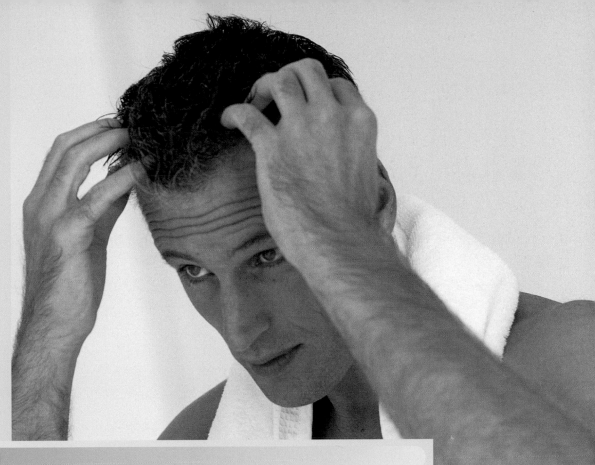

styling

Just as for women, a good cut can make you look like a Pierce Brosnan doppelganger, while a bad one can add years on and/or make you invisible. Here are six tips to help you make the most of your hair:

1   Don't ignore your style. What worked twenty years ago is no good now. Fashions change (even in men's hair) and your hair texture and needs are unlikely to stay the same forever. You need an update if you haven't changed style in three years.

2   Avoid long hair (especially if it is thinning or balding) and, most of all, avoid long hair tied back in a ponytail – it is a real turn-off.

3   Avoid hair all one length. If it is thick, you will look like Michael Heseltine or Melvyn Bragg. Even Hugh Grant has had a haircut and doesn't he look better now? If it is thin, it will be flyaway and messy. Get it razor-cut and/or cut into shaggy layers you can mess up a little with some gel and look quite subtly trendy.

4   If you need to look smart and formal, the cut just mentioned can also look that way if you blow-dry it with a small brush and use a little leave-in conditioner.

5   Make sure your hairdresser bears in mind your head and face shapes when choosing a new cut. Even small changes can make all the difference. For example, if you have a low forehead (not much space between brows and hair-line) and/or a large, long jaw, you need the hair taken off the brow and up to balance out the face shape; with a high forehead, a shaggy fringe can look great.

6   Don't be afraid to use products to improve condition, shine, manageability and the range of styles you can make within one cut (see Styling products, page 151).

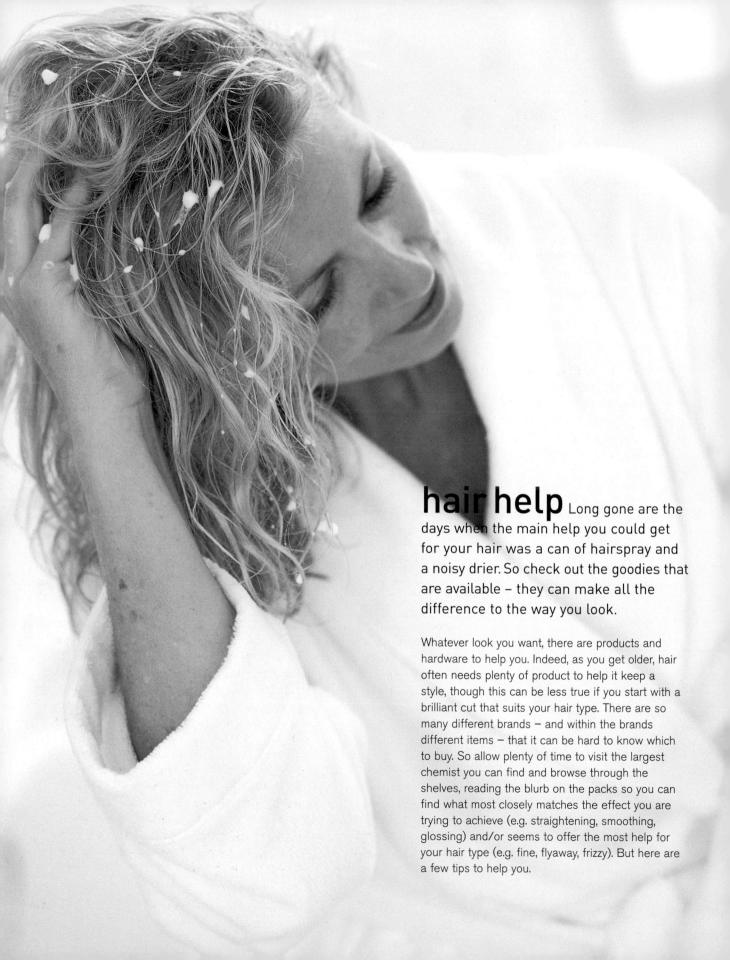

hair help

Long gone are the days when the main help you could get for your hair was a can of hairspray and a noisy drier. So check out the goodies that are available – they can make all the difference to the way you look.

Whatever look you want, there are products and hardware to help you. Indeed, as you get older, hair often needs plenty of product to help it keep a style, though this can be less true if you start with a brilliant cut that suits your hair type. There are so many different brands – and within the brands different items – that it can be hard to know which to buy. So allow plenty of time to visit the largest chemist you can find and browse through the shelves, reading the blurb on the packs so you can find what most closely matches the effect you are trying to achieve (e.g. straightening, smoothing, glossing) and/or seems to offer the most help for your hair type (e.g. fine, flyaway, frizzy). But here are a few tips to help you.

styling products

Makers of styling products have lately developed an extraordinary range of names, but basically they can be grouped into just a few categories.

Leave-in conditioners, which you work in or spray in after you've finished washing and have towel-dried your hair. They can be used after, or instead of, ordinary rinse-out conditioner, depending on how dry your hair is. There are leave-ins for all hair types, so choose carefully. They are particularly useful if you are going to use hot hardware on or near your hair, as they help prevent over-drying. If you tend towards greasy, limp hair, you may be better off avoiding these conditioners and choosing a blow-dry lotion instead.

Styling mousse or volumizer is good for adding control and volume to fine, flyaway and limp hair without added 'grease'.

Styling gels, clays and waxes are good for short styles with a modern look – tousled or spiky, for instance. Combined with a decent cut, they can take years off you. For curly styles without frizz, there are serums that you run through wet hair.

Glossers are usually poured into your palm and spread evenly through the hair once you have styled it, to add gloss and a healthy look. In my experience, they are best used on ends only and in small quantity.

Hairspray is still around, but better than it used to be. It can help you avoid that flyaway look without (if you pick carefully) being too 'set'.

shampoos, conditioners and colour savers

All-in-one shampoo/conditioners have fallen out of favour in recent years, but one or two brands are still available and are ideal if you really are in a hurry.

Shampoos are best bought in trial sizes or sachets, if available, because what it says on the bottle can only give you a general idea of whether or not that particular brand will suit your hair. Price isn't always an indication of quality either.

Conditioners often work best if teamed with a shampoo in the same brand range, and conditioning creams should be avoided if your hair is thin, limp or greasy. For longer hair, condition the bottom half only. Sixty per cent of us colour our hair, and for us the new colour-saving shampoos and conditioners may be a good idea – if you are fair, the Sheer Blonde range is definitely for you.

colorants

If you've never coloured your hair before, start out with a temporary colour based on vegetable dye, then move to a semi-permanent, which lasts about six weeks, and finally, when you're sure, a permanent (or stick with the semi for a colour look that fades more naturally rather than giving you a 'grow-out' line). Today you can even get a kit that you can use to give yourself highlights, so you don't need to visit the hairdresser if you hate that 'solid' block of colour that home-colouring always used to give. If you are trying to cover grey, you will need a permanent, and pick a brand produced especially for the purpose.

Home colours can rarely help you go more than two shades lighter than your natural colour without bleach-type lightening, so if it is a blonde look you want, you are best off visiting a good colourist.

hardware

Even if it takes you a few tries to produce professional-looking results with equipment that seemed so easy at the hairdresser's, it is worth investing in some up-to-date hair hardware.

Older hair can become drier and more flyaway, in which case a combination of a light leave-in conditioner and straightening tongs (for a dead straight look) or a drier with a built-in smoothing brush (for a smooth look with a little more volume and curve to it) should work well. Straighteners have either metal plates or ceramic ones – professionals say that ceramics are kinder on the hair and produce better results. Don't bother buying a straightener with a steam facility, which is unwieldy and prevents you getting the tongs close to your scalp. Straighten your hair instead when it is still slightly damp, for an even better result. Dull hair always looks much more glossy when you use a straightener, as it smooths down the hair cuticles and reflects more light.

If you have curly longish hair, a diffuser drier used with serum is still one of the best options, as it removes the risk of frizz and flyaway. If you have wavy or straight hair that you want to curl, get curling tongs with at least three different size attachments and, as the heat is direct on the hair and is held without moving for several seconds (unlike with a straightener, where the tongs keep moving over the hair), it is very important to use a conditioning style aid before beginning to use the curling tongs.

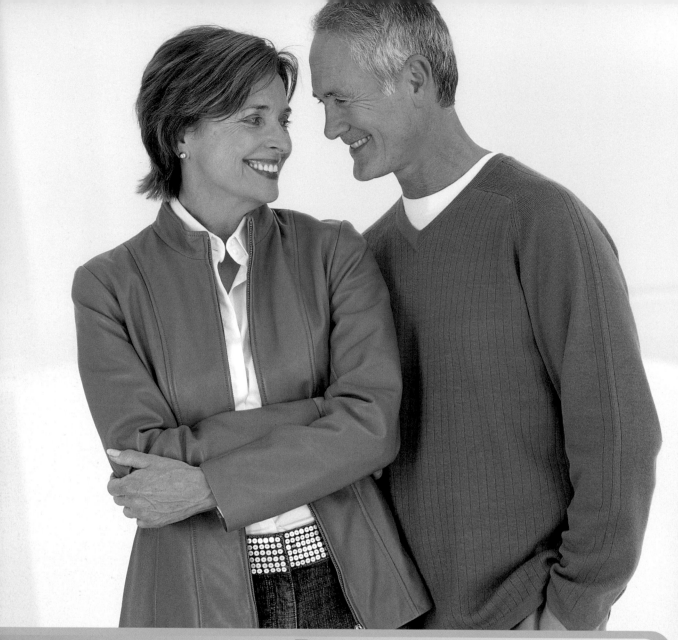

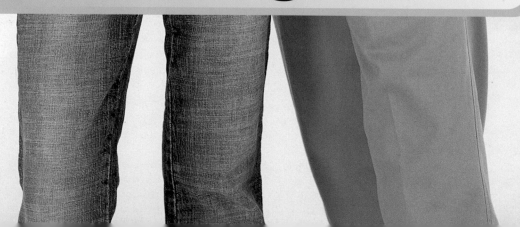

repackage yourself

Clothes say who you are – or who you want to be. They can make people believe in you, take notice of you … and have you believe in yourself. So don't fade away … begin finding a wardrobe that suits your needs today. **packaging sells** Your packaging is the clothes that you choose every day - and learning to 'market' yourself by what you wear is a vital part of a new mid-life image. You need to look great, whether the look for you today is smart, casual, chic, glam or country...

If you look good, it is easier to sell yourself to new people. First impressions count. Within a few seconds of meeting you, new contacts – such as prospective employers, potential lovers – will decide whether you fit in with their image of what they are looking for, will gauge your age, will probably even guess at your income, your social status and your IQ. And a large percentage of these assumptions will be based on what you are wearing.

If you know that the clothes you wear – not only for special occasions but also on an everyday basis – project the image of you that YOU want to project, then you feel confident and you WILL do better in life. That image doesn't have to be 'power', it can be gentle, feminine, masculine, relaxed, dynamic …whatever you want it to be. And research shows that if you present your desirable image, even if you don't feel that way at first, you soon will. For example, you're feeling sad and lonely, but you go to an event wearing a 'look at me' red dress and soon you're living the 'carefree, centre of attention' role you project.

In other words, clothes also help you sell yourself to YOU. They can help lift any negative emotions, while, if they make you look fat, dowdy, old-fashioned, tired, bedraggled, too young, too old or uncomfortable, then they will make you feel worse. Look good – and suddenly you feel YES! I have possibilities; I still have a life.

Even if you are doing nothing more than spending a day at home, relaxing and reading the papers, your clothes can help you to feel good. Huge rewards can be had for a small outlay of time and cash. Worth doing? YES.

So WHAT to do? Repackaging yourself needn't take a great deal of time or even money, but you need to know what you want to achieve, so it does take thought and research. DO you need a total revamp? New ideas for home, work, evenings, holidays? What do you want to spend? You also need to know what dressing right for your age really means.

dressing for your shape – women
We all have features that we don't like, or imperfections in our shape. And however much you look after your body via diet and exercise, as you age you can expect to see changes to your shape. The tips here should help you to choose clothes that minimize the less good points and maximize the best.

tall and skinny?
Lucky you! You can wear almost anything and look elegant – which is why catwalk models are all ultra-tall and thin. Make the most of your looks by going with all the looks that plumper women can't wear – such as clingy cashmere, slightly cropped tops, boxy jackets, blousons and thick tweeds for autumn and winter, and flowing chiffons, florals and ethnic looks for summer. Long skirts and flatties like Birkenstocks or ballet pumps look great all year round and, if you really don't like your swan neck, long scarves which break up the outline of what you are wearing do the trick. If you really do want to look shorter (why?), choose separates in differing shades, rather than an all-in-one look.

short?
Oh, the delight of being able to wear high heels without towering over anyone! But don't wear them TOO tall with skirts, or you will simply look ridiculous (with trousers that nearly touch the floor, they are fine). Shop at stores which cater specially for petite sizes so that the fit of what you buy will be good. Go for fitted looks which will flatter rather than swamp you, and aim for a long line of colour rather than breaking the look up. Shift dresses and coat and suit dresses rather than jacket and trousers, for example. Stick with small accessories – jewellery, belts, hats – and small prints or plains.

large bust?
There is no way you can ignore your bust by hiding it under voluminous tops so you really do need to 'go with it'. First you need to kit yourself out with some good-quality supporting and flattering bras which lift your bust off your waist and give you a cleavage, then you need to choose clothes that give a shape to your waist and hips, to create the hour-glass figure. To do this you may need to buy separates, as your bust may be a bigger size than your waist/hips and you DON'T want any top that is too tight. A V-neck is much better than a high neck. Avoid short jackets and go for well-tailored longer lengths, slightly fitted. If you have slim legs, go for shorter skirts and high heels.

no waist?
Best to go for the androgynous look, with well-tailored trouser suits (there are many good makes that have surreptitiously elasticated panels in the sides to allow for a couple of extra inches) for more formal wear. Hipster jeans can be a surprisingly good idea, if they are not too tight, as they sit below the waist. Coupled with a blouson top or well-cut shirt, they can disguise a large waist very well. Any dress or tunic that skims the waist is good – avoid belted dresses and skirts, and particularly avoid gathers and pleats.

If you have a large waist, you've probably got slim thighs (the apple shape), so show them off in boot-cuts and shortish skirts (mini depending on age).

fat tum?
Without saying the 'corset' word, it is true that if you have a tum that sticks out or wobbles somewhat, while the rest of you is pretty OK, then – until you have the sit-ups licked – some supportive underwear is a fine substitute – available from any good department store (try before you buy). You don't have to be ultra-constricted these days to feel nicely helped around your middle.

Avoid clingy tops and any lines that finish on the stomach (e.g. a short boxy jacket or cardigan) and avoid straight skirts or any skirts with a waist-band that will show. Also avoid anything tucked into the waistband, and instead go for skimming looks or blousons. Black or navy 'absorb' a fat tum and eye-catching detail around the bust and neckline also help

big hips or thighs?

You need to remember two things — first, balance your shape out by wearing tailored tops with strong shoulder lines or Ts, jumpers, etc. with wide necklines; second, take the eye away from the hips and the thighs by choosing muted colours for both your trousers and skirts, and brights, pastels or patterns for the top, as well as big-statement jewellery or scarves, for instance. If you have a good bust, a deep V or scoop neck may also be a good idea.

It also helps to avoid any jackets or tops that finish on the widest part of your hips or thighs, and go for trousers in thin material either straight-legged or slightly flared. Leather and suede will add inches to your hips — avoid them.

large?

There are two main mistakes many bigger women make when they choose clothes. One, they dress in what they feel is disguise, using baggy clothes and loose fits. This absolutely doesn't work — such clothes actually make you look fatter. Otherwise, they choose one size too small (or continue to wear their old, thinner wardrobe) in the hope that this will also act as a disguise. Straining zips and buttons and rolls of fat don't work, though.

The only way to dress if you are over-weight is in good-quality clothes. Sharp tailoring, which skims over your fatter bits, can make you look two stone slimmer. Dark colours can work well, but — with the right cut — so can lights and neutrals. Matt materials absorb weight, shiny materials accentuate them. Consider 'plus' size designers and stores, some of which are excellent.

Every woman has some best bits — for example, if you are plump you may have very young-looking skin and face … show them off with light colours around the face and a great haircut..

for men

short
go for fitted styles, single-breasted jackets and suits, pinstripes, suits all one colour rather than trousers with a differently coloured top, shoes with a small heel.
avoid double breasted suits, turn-ups on trousers.

narrow shoulders/ skinny arms
go for tailored jackets (made-to-measure will be a great investment), blouson-style leather jackets, generously tailored shirts.
avoid V-neck sweaters (in fact, most sweaters), skimpy T-shirts (especially coupled with baggy trousers), vest tops, raglan sleeves.

wide
go for dark, single-breasted jackets or suits teamed with similarly coloured shirts and ties, or pale/bold shirts and ties, very good-quality tailoring which skims not clings.
avoid jeans, combats (which can be narrow at the ankle and will make you look ever wider), double - breasted jackets and coats.

pot
go for trousers cut with a slightly low waist and plenty of room around the waist and hips (tightly cut trousers just accentuate your belly), hip-skimming jackets, roomy dark-coloured sweaters.
avoid tight jeans and trousers, hipsters (belly sags over belt – horrible); clingy T-shirts, shirts that button too tight over the belly, double-breasted suits.

top 10 ways to avoid the timewarp trap

Nothing gives away your age quicker than a wardrobe that is years out of date or stuck in a particular era. Use these tips to get yourself up to date and younger-looking without being MODAL (mutton obviously dressed as lamb).

1 Shop regularly – i.e. at least twice a year for main items of clothing and 4 times a year for small pieces. That way you're bound to stay up to date. If you're not near a good selection of shops, don't forget the Internet and catalogues – or treat yourself to a weekend shopping trip with a friend.

2 Buy one or two fashion magazines a month – *Vogue*, *Harpers*, *In Style*, *Red* - for general ideas and direction. Don't just read the editorial, look at the adverts too, which will give you ideas on which stores have the kind of clothes you would like and in which you would feel comfortable.

3 Enlist help if you are frightened of change. Whose look do you most admire amongst your friends or family? Ask them to shop with you or, if you can afford it, have a personal shopper (available at many department stores) to help and advise you. A freelance personal stylist might not be a huge extravagance once or twice in a lifetime. Try on things even if you think they won't suit you.

4 Always remember that the clothes you loved ten years ago are highly unlikely ever to be lovely again. Lifestyles change, we change, fashions change, bodies change. Chuck out anything in your wardrobe that's more than three years old and which you haven't worn in that time – unless it is a true vintage piece, which can be cleaned and kept in a bag in storage, or sold. And chuck out anything older than five years, even if you have worn it in that time, except vintage ditto. Think of your wardrobe as a larder, with clothes each having their use-by date.

5 Look at photographs of yourself five and ten years ago. Is your style evolving or do you look alarmingly similar now to how you did then?

6 Get in the habit of looking at what other people are wearing when you are on the train, in the office, in shops, socializing. Become a fashion critic. What looks good, what doesn't – and why? Trinny and Susannah didn't go to uni to learn about style – you can do it too. Apply what you see to yourself.

7 And get in the habit of each day giving your outfit a critical once-over in a full-length mirror. Allow yourself time to get dressed and to decide what looks good and what doesn't.

8 Twice a year, buy a few accessories – scarves, hats, gloves, jewellery – in this season's colours (or those of them that you like). These will immediately update your wardrobe of more basic colours.

9 If you wear glasses, update them every year or, at the least, two. Fashions in frame styles and colours alter frequently and, if you are still wearing frames from years ago, they will immediately date you. Choose an optician with a large range and devote at least half an hour to trying on as many as you can. Don't just go for something you like the look of – make sure they suit your face. Suitable frames can actually improve your looks. Tinted and/or reactolite lenses can also look cool.

10 Even if you can't afford to update major clothes every season, a new pair of shoes or boots in an up-to-the minute style will make the whole outfit look more now.

rethink your wardrobe
Once you've read the preceding pages you may have a clearer idea of how you need to revamp your wardrobe. Use the images on the following pages to give you ideas. Men, please turn to page 164.

'I want to look younger'
See Top 10 Ways to Avoid the Time Warp Trap opposite, which should help you to dress to suit yourself without looking too old or, even worse, too young.

Remember also that colouring of both skin and hair change over the years and that, as you get older, paler and warmer colours, such as cream, beige and apricot, may make you look younger than harder blacks, greys or blues.

'I want casual but smart'
There will always be a place for blue jeans and T-shirts in our lives, but sometimes it is good to wear other types of casuals. Similarly, while you may be used to wearing a suit to work, you might just as easily wear something less formal without sacrificing smartness.

The key to 'smart casual' is choosing good-quality clothes which fit you very well, and think Gucci rather than Dorothy Perkins when accessorizing. The most relaxed of outfits can be smartened with the addition of a well-cut jacket. Also remember that ultra-casual styles can appear smart if they are made in a 'smart' fabric, such as suede, tweed, silk or linen. In general, avoid the tackier end of man-made fibres, going for at least a mix that contains 80% natural fibre.

'I want to wear funky clothes'
Well, it's partly in the definition. Are we talking Zandra or Dolly Parton? Madonna or Pam Anderson? You also need confidence in your own sense of style. You need to buy and wear something because that is what you really want, and that is what you want to say about yourself. The chosen items should also fall happily into your lifestyle. Up to a point, you have to dress to suit what your life is, rather than what it was or what it might be in your memory or imagination. That said, there is rarely any harm in being bold at any age.

'I want to show flesh'
(see page 163) This isn't an age thing so much as a body thing. Daily workouts with weights and lucky skin may mean that at 40 or 50 you can show acres of flesh with pride. However, if not acres, most of us can at least show a tantalizing glimpse .

'I want to look sexy'
(see page 162) Sexy dressing means different things to different people. Some, for instance, are attracted to under-stated sexiness – a complete cover-up with a hint of gorgeous figure underneath, perhaps – while others think sexy equals skin-tight mini-skirted Lycra.

I want to wear brights'
(see page 160) There's no need to put on the brown, or even the baby pink, just because you hit 50. Try on lots of stuff before you buy and begin with small splashes of colour. Alternatively, if you've always worn brights and now wonder whether they are still OK, take your favourite colours (scarves are good for this), hold them up in daylight against your face and see if they flatter or make you look washed out.

'I want to look good on a budget'
(overleaf) Very easy today – thanks to discount villages, chain stores such as TK Maxx, and regular sales at the major designer boutiques (Addresses, page 236). Even the least expensive clothes can look great if you choose well and wash and dry them carefully. TIP: Cheaper clothes tend to be cut smaller.

'I want classic with a twist'
(see page 159) Classic styles can look very good, but if you spent years in the chain fashion stores before deciding you need to dress more like a 40-year-old than a 20-year-old, you might find the classic high-street looks and/or the older designers boring – they might make you feel old. Seek out the classics that have their own edge – like Armani, Betty Jackson, Dolce e Gabbana.

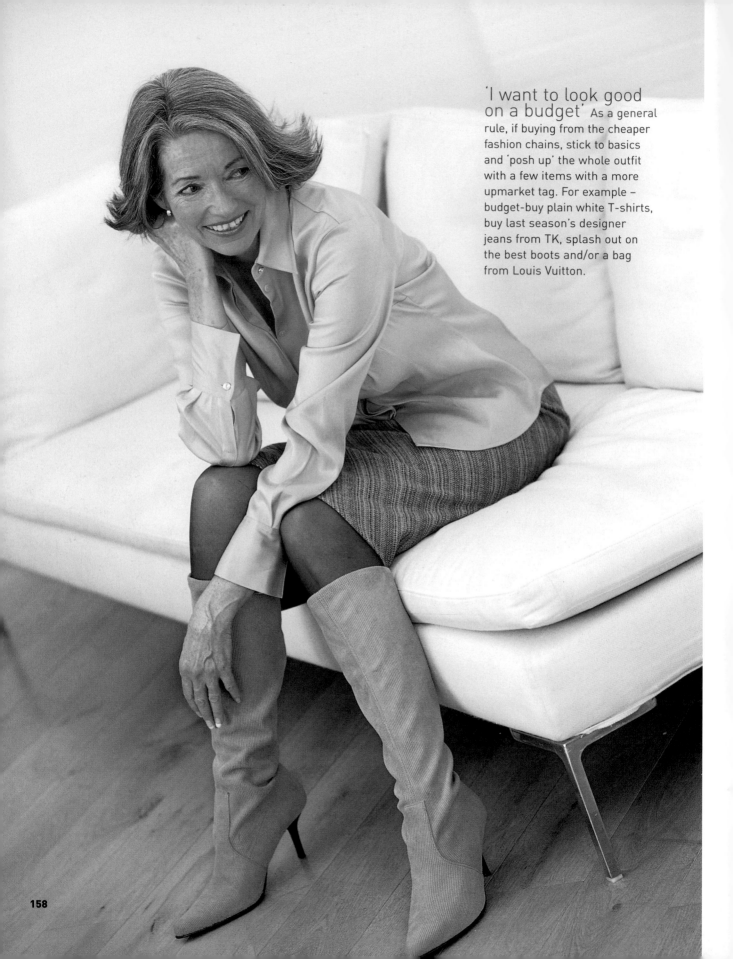

'I want to look good on a budget' As a general rule, if buying from the cheaper fashion chains, stick to basics and 'posh up' the whole outfit with a few items with a more upmarket tag. For example – budget-buy plain white T-shirts, buy last season's designer jeans from TK, splash out on the best boots and/or a bag from Louis Vuitton.

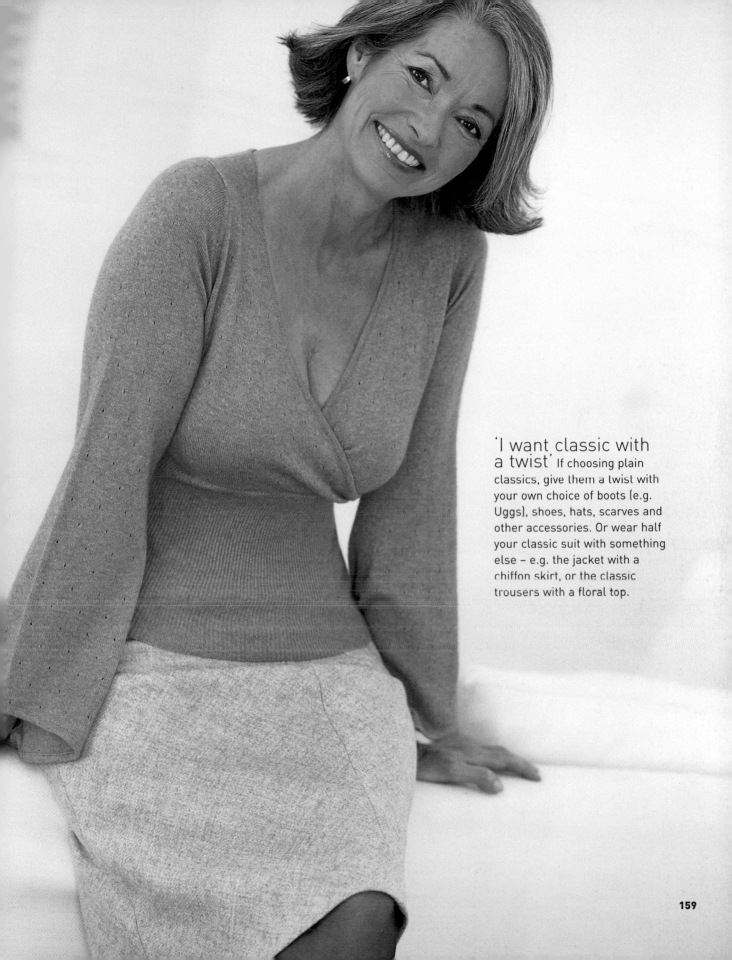

'I want classic with a twist' If choosing plain classics, give them a twist with your own choice of boots (e.g. Uggs), shoes, hats, scarves and other accessories. Or wear half your classic suit with something else – e.g. the jacket with a chiffon skirt, or the classic trousers with a floral top.

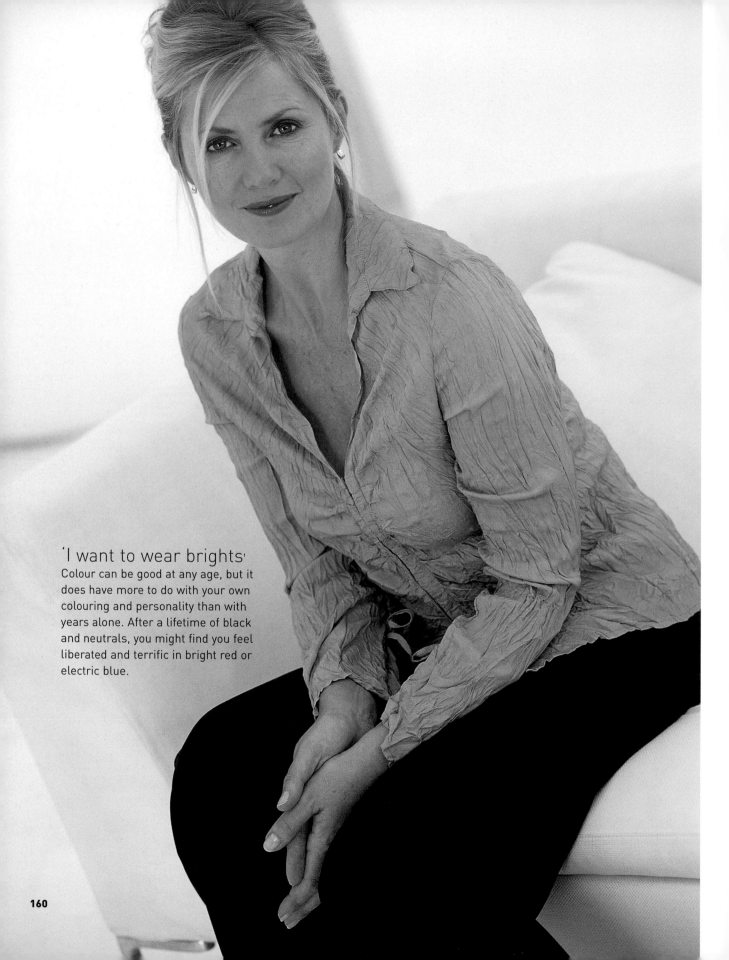

'I want to wear brights'

Colour can be good at any age, but it does have more to do with your own colouring and personality than with years alone. After a lifetime of black and neutrals, you might find you feel liberated and terrific in bright red or electric blue.

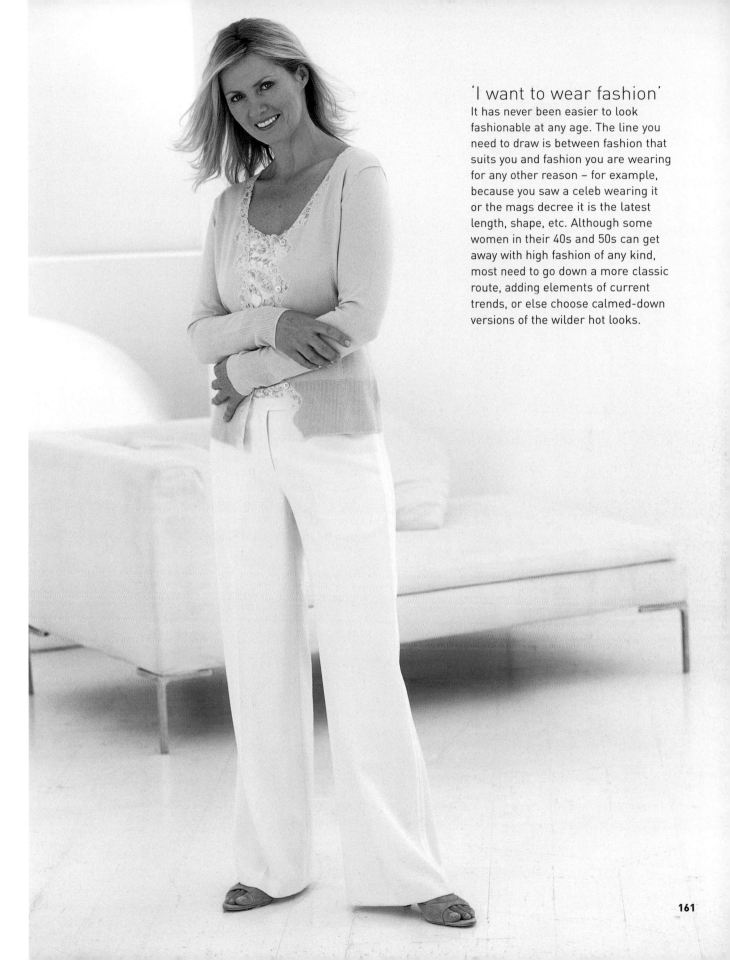

'I want to wear fashion'

It has never been easier to look fashionable at any age. The line you need to draw is between fashion that suits you and fashion you are wearing for any other reason – for example, because you saw a celeb wearing it or the mags decree it is the latest length, shape, etc. Although some women in their 40s and 50s can get away with high fashion of any kind, most need to go down a more classic route, adding elements of current trends, or else choose calmed-down versions of the wilder hot looks.

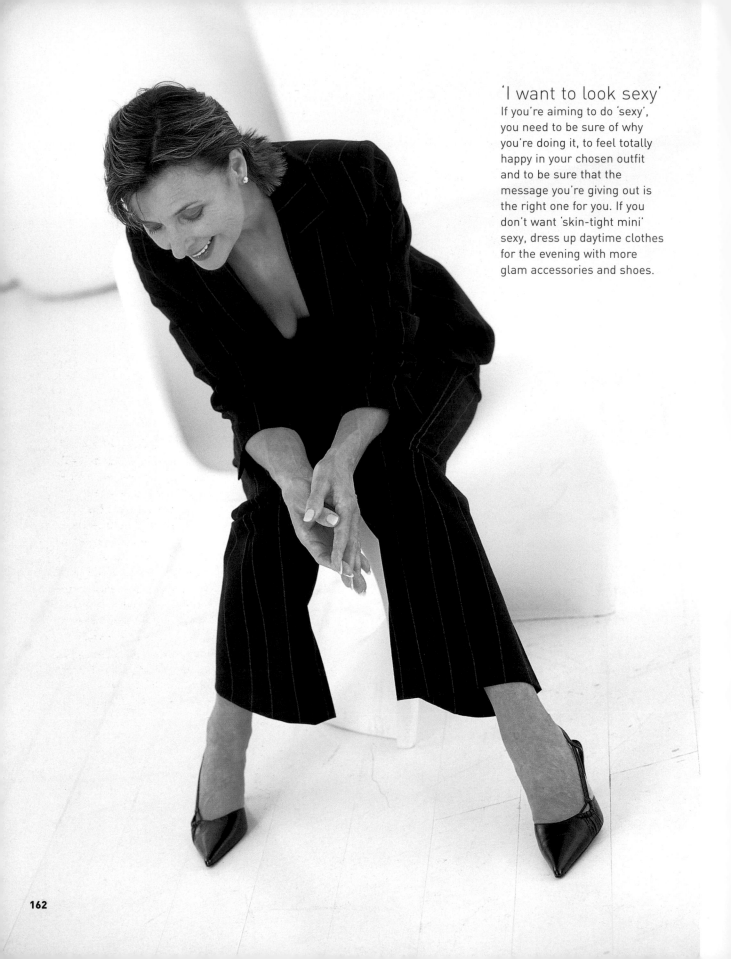

'I want to look sexy'
If you're aiming to do 'sexy', you need to be sure of why you're doing it, to feel totally happy in your chosen outfit and to be sure that the message you're giving out is the right one for you. If you don't want 'skin-tight mini' sexy, dress up daytime clothes for the evening with more glam accessories and shoes.

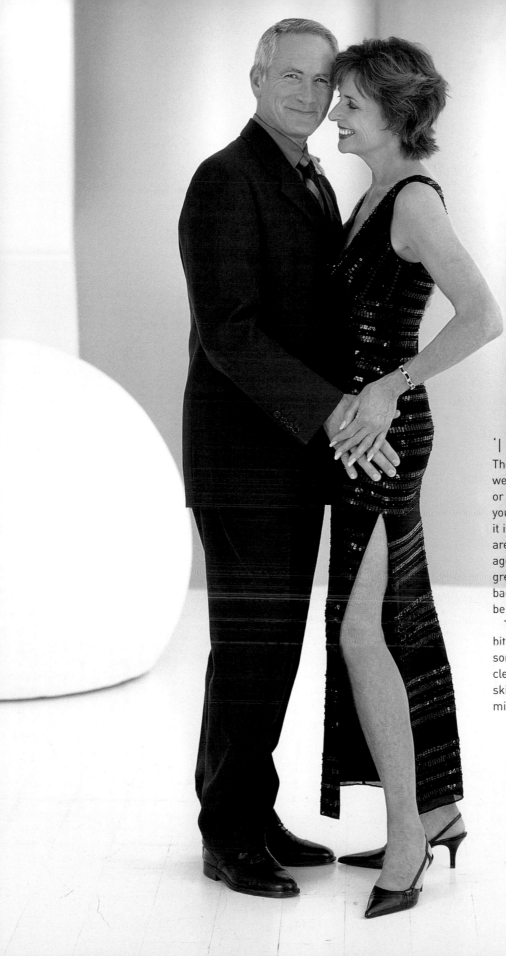

'I want to show flesh'

There's no reason why you can't wear a miniskirt in the summer, or split skirt in the evening, if you have fabulous legs (which, it is always said patronizingly, are the 'last things to go' as we age!). Cleavage can also be great. And take a look at your back in the mirror – it may well be worth showing off.

The best rule is that for every bit of flesh you show, cover something else up. For example, cleavage on display equals long skirt and/or long sleeves; miniskirt equals polo neck.

and for men If your idea of taking a fashion risk is buying a sweatshirt in the sales, take time to bring new life into your wardrobe.

It is said that 35% of British men aged over 45 never set foot inside a male boutique or shop, feeling that fashion is for females and that someone else will shop for them if there is an emergency (weight gain renders complete wardrobe useless; everything has fallen to pieces in the wash; wedding or job interview to attend).

And yet … if a man does have a proper makeover, he always ends up with a bashful grin of real delight. 'I DO look good!' 'I COULD still play the game!' Just one day of your life is all it might take to achieve near miracles, so if you want to give it a try, here's a six-point plan:

1 Go through your existing wardrobe (I won't use the word 'current' as it probably isn't) and be ruthless, trying things on if necessary. Put into a bin bag everything that is old, tired-looking, out of shape, bedraggled, worn, stained, shrunk, discoloured. In the bag also goes anything that is unflattering (try on!) for you in shape (see page 155), colour, material or in any other way. Ditto everything that is too tight, too small, too short – the only possible exception is if you are currently losing weight.

If there is anything left, sort it through and chuck out what is dated – although men's fashion moves slowly, over five years old and it needs binning (classically tailored top-quality suits and jackets excepted). Anyway, you need a change, don't you?

Lastly, discard anything that is too teenage or too dotage for you. Put it on. Do you look like you're trying to be your son? Or your father? If not sure, ask your partner. Take the bags immediately to the dump so that you aren't tempted to put everything back.

2 List your purchase priorities according to your lifestyle (Mostly casual? Work? Sporting? Home wear? Travel?) and what is left in your wardrobe.

This could be a new suit, 2–3 shirts, 3 ties, 2 heavyweight sweaters, 2 lightweight cotton sweaters, 2 pairs of smart casual trousers, I pair of jeans, 3 T-shirts, 2 pairs of shoes, 2 belts.

Bear in mind the current season and, if you can't afford to buy a lot, buy half this season (spring/summer or autumn/winter) and half the next. This will also help you keep up to date.

3 Take your measurements (with help): neck, chest, waist, hips, inner leg. Write them down.

4 Decide where, when and how to shop. Nothing beats trying things on, so real shops are preferable to mail order or Internet (although, of course, you can return unsuitable items and these methods can be good for some people). Department stores are usually good on range of prices, labels and styles, and if you are an uncomfortable or virgin shopper, smaller boutiques and shops can be daunting. Some larger stores offer the assistance of a personal shopper, which may be free or you may pay a fee (usually well worth it). Or, take an acquaintance with a good sense of style who knows you well.

5 Armed with your shopping list and your size list, shop. Set aside a minimum of several hours to do your shopping and try hard to make sure that your chosen pieces coordinate with each other, so that you will look smarter and you can mix and match.

6 Begin wearing your new clothes straight away – they aren't to be saved for a rainy day. And remember now to shop AT LEAST once a year. It's only fashion … but you know you like it really.

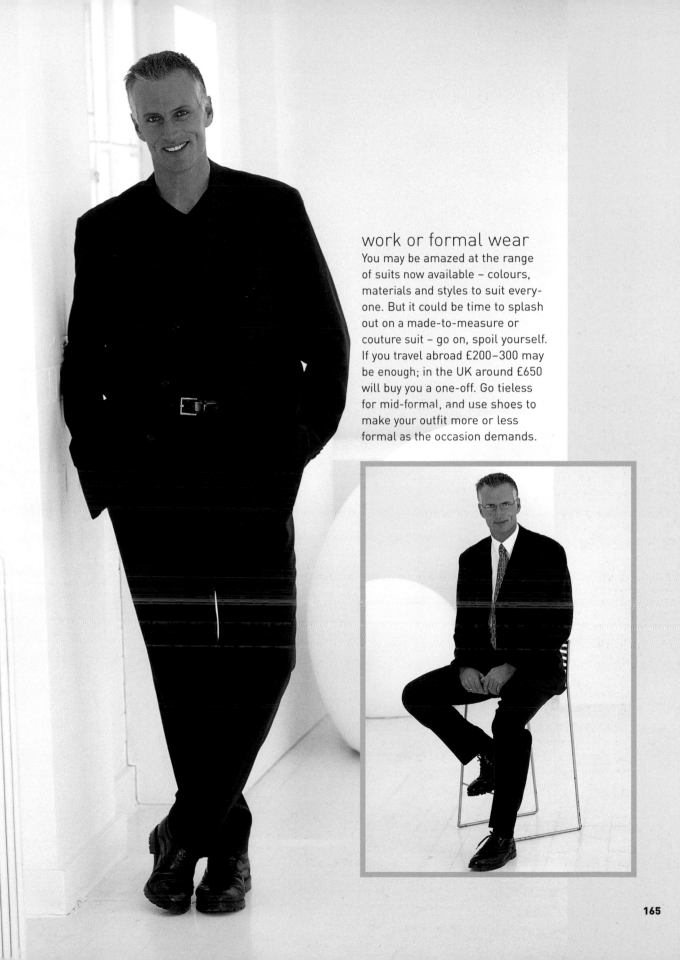

work or formal wear

You may be amazed at the range of suits now available – colours, materials and styles to suit everyone. But it could be time to splash out on a made-to-measure or couture suit – go on, spoil yourself. If you travel abroad £200–300 may be enough; in the UK around £650 will buy you a one-off. Go tieless for mid-formal, and use shoes to make your outfit more or less formal as the occasion demands.

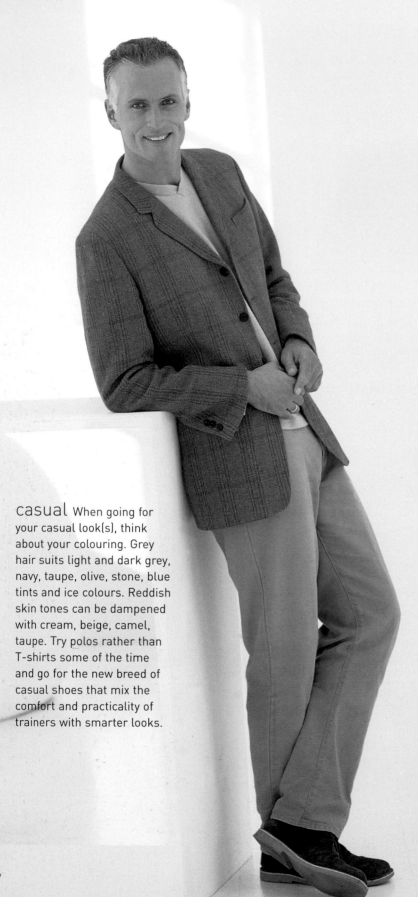

jeans for men

Many times I have heard it said that people over 50 (sometimes even 40) shouldn't wear jeans – and yet they are a mainstay of nearly everyone's wardrobe, whatever your age, male or female. Men, in particular, would be lost without their denims ... So if you've ever had anyone sneer a little at your post-40 body in your Levi's, here are some tips to bear in mind:

● Buy a new pair of blue jeans at least once a year – only pre-25s can get away with rips and fraying, without looking like a homeless person.

● Pay attention to cut. If you have a large belly, choose jeans with a slight flare. Avoid hipsters unless you have a perfect figure. Don't buy them too tight on the leg unless you have a perfect figure, with long, lean legs.

● Dark denim looks better as you get older.

● Try something new – jeans in black denim are smart and, teamed with a good jacket or well-cut shirt, can take you almost anywhere.

● All jeans look much smarter if worn with a good-quality leather belt.

● Don't wear trainers with your jeans all the time ... loafers can look terrific and expensive leather can smarten up any colour of jeans.

● Avoid white socks. Wear either no socks (summer) or socks to match your jeans or shoes.

casual When going for your casual look(s), think about your colouring. Grey hair suits light and dark grey, navy, taupe, olive, stone, blue tints and ice colours. Reddish skin tones can be dampened with cream, beige, camel, taupe. Try polos rather than T-shirts some of the time and go for the new breed of casual shoes that mix the comfort and practicality of trainers with smarter looks.

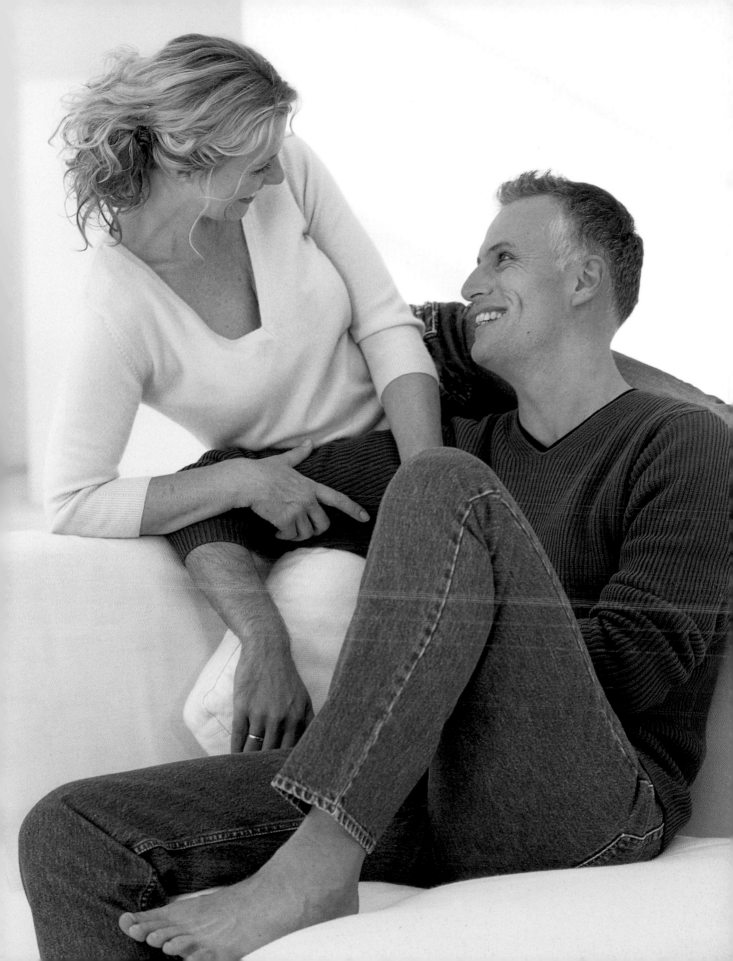

well-being
for your
newlife

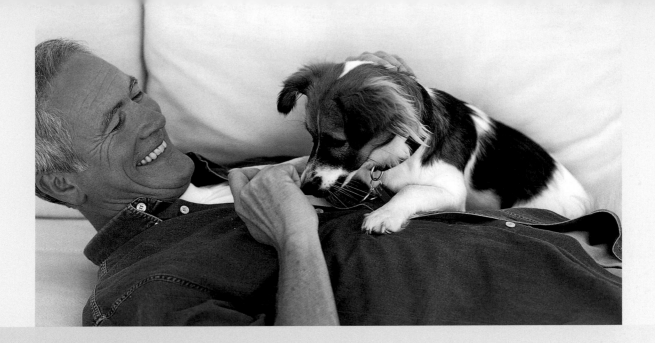

With few exceptions, life is as good as YOU feel ... research shows that good health can improve not only your physical and mental capabilities but also your appearance and your outlook. So if you want to enjoy yourself, not only in the present but also for the rest of your days, it is vital to look after yourself.

True good health comes from a holistic approach, and in this section we look at all the aspects of well-being that particularly affect people in mid life. From the female menopause and male andropause, and the sexual dilemmas that many people face at this time, through to problems such as tiredness, depression and stress, and on to the life-threatening diseases like cancer and diabetes, in Section 4 you will find the inspiration – and the answers – to help you make mid life your healthiest time yet.

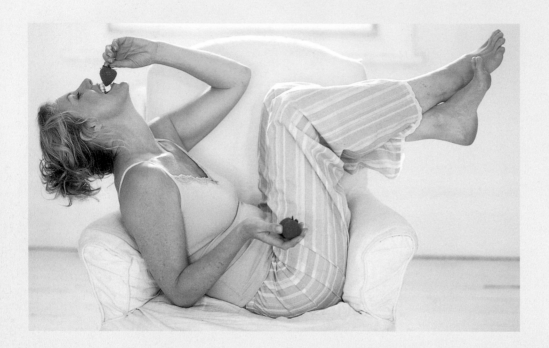

if you take some care now, you can live not only a longer life, but also one that gives you more independence, enjoyment, contentment, excitement and so on.

While a hundred years ago you were likely to end your life at around the age of 50, in the twenty-first century mid-lifers can expect to live on for at least another thirty years, with unprecedented numbers of men and women now also reaching their 90s and the magic 100-plus.

Even better news is that, according to US research, the period of 'old age' (with ill health and disability) is becoming shorter and shorter, so that our 'middle age' now extends to at least the age of 70.

In other words – despite all the doom and gloom and health scares – you can probably look forward to a long and healthy life ahead of you even if you are already into your 50s or 60s. HOWEVER, to maximize this potential, you do need to look after yourself.

Section 4 is all about making the most of what you have, healthwise, and minimizing the problems. For women the major physical 'event' of mid life is the menopause. We look at what actually happens, the pros and cons of HRT and alternative treatments. And it is not just women who are affected by physical changes in mid life.

At this time, it is common for the libido to diminish, and a poor sex life can spoil the best of relationships. The second chapter in the section answers questions such as, 'What is normal?' 'What can be done to overcome libido problems in both men and women?' Poor libido may often be caused by the health problems that are common in mid life, and in the chapter that follows we examine these. One of the major cries I hear is 'I am tired/exhausted/ have no energy.' Although a frequent problem, lack of energy and sparkle is not insurmountable, so we look at solutions, including how to get a good night's sleep.

Body aches and pains can be a depressing and debilitating arrival in mid life. We examine how to manage – or even largely avoid – arthritis and other muscular/skeletal problems, and look at what – apart from diet and exercise (already discussed) – can be done to protect your bones against osteoporosis.

Many people over 45 or so tell me that they can no longer take for granted that their digestive system will operate smoothly and without complaint. Irritable bowel, ulcers and heartburn are three 'spoilers' that can all be contained, as you will see. If you want to live a long and healthy life, you need to minimize your risk of getting one of the 'big three' diseases of middle age – heart disease, cancer and diabetes. You also need to consider your intake of alcohol, possibly tackle a nicotine habit and even get to grips with your intake of drugs – whether they are over-the-counter, prescribed or illegal! Giving up a habit is easier than you might think...

Lastly, you can find help for your state of mind. Anxiety, depression, stress and poor memory are all common in mid life, but they can be tackled and controlled. Well-being is what you can have, and what you need, if you are to also enjoy the great benefits of those later mid-life years ... time, freedom and independence.

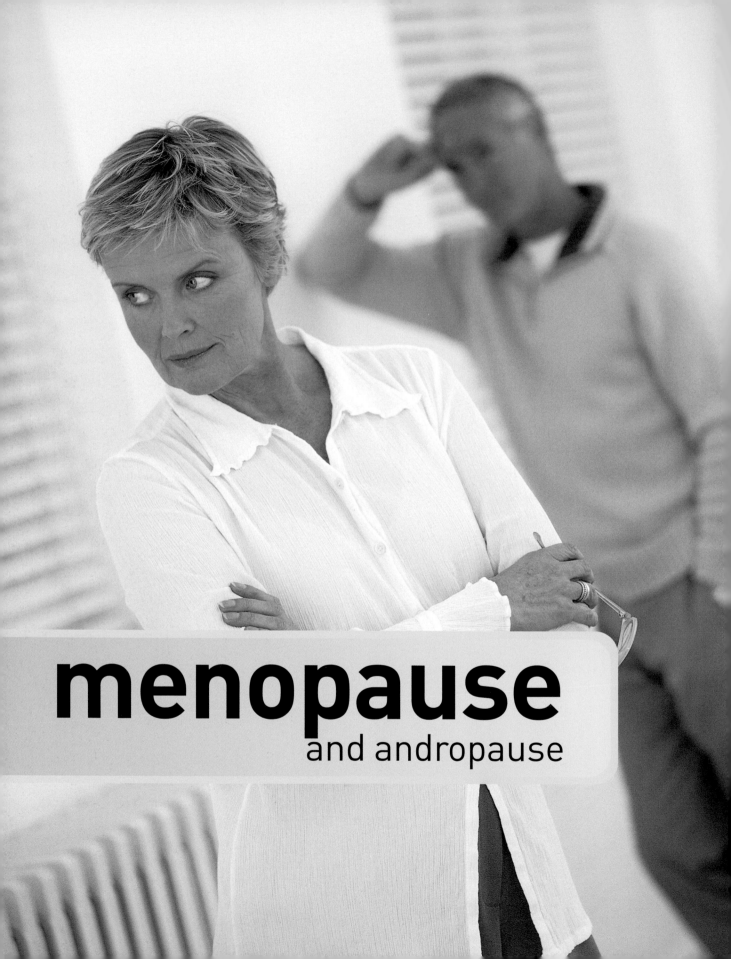

menopause
and andropause

In their late 40s or early 50s, most women (and many men) go through far-reaching changes, both physical and emotional. If you understand and manage what is happening to you, the menopausal/andropausal years – and those that follow – can be a change for the better.

Most women begin the peri-menopause in their late forties, with periods becoming erratic, which leads – on average by the age of 51 – to the menopause itself, when periods and reproductive life cease.

The male menopause is a much-debated topic, with many professionals believing that it doesn't exist, but very many men are quite convinced that it certainly does. Men may not have periods to lose, but they can testify that night sweats, hot flushes, lack of libido and other annoying symptoms most definitely do happen.

We look at the side-effects of both male and female menopause and see how best you can cope during this time which, let's face it, is a big chunk out of your life. If you ask doctors how long your symptoms, like hot flushes, will last, most will say three to four years. In truth, however, they can last for much longer than that, and often do.

We also discuss the long-term effects that going through the 'change', as it is sometimes called, may bring. There is much research indicating that after the menopause women are more susceptible to illnesses such as heart disease and breast cancer. Many women put on a lot of weight in these years, though some scientists still believe there is no hormonal link causing this to happen. Most people are also aware that, when periods cease, bone loss accelerates and this can lead to the debilitating disease osteoporosis.

Over the past 30 years or more, hormone replacement therapy (HRT) has been heralded as the complete answer to beating menopausal symptoms in women, and lowering the long-term health risks. In recent years, however, there has been a move away from HRT, after fears that it could cause its own health problems. We look at the facts, and also at the many alternative natural and herbal remedies on offer. They may be natural – but do they work? While for men, are there ANY remedies they can buy for their own andropausal symptoms?

Amidst all this uncertainty and confusion, what is certain is that most people do find ways to survive, with their sanity intact, and agree that life is as good as ever, during the menopausal years and after.

facts about the menopause Many of us have
little or no conception of what happens before and during the menopause. Here we look
at what it really means.

women

The phase leading up to the female menopause, which often begins in the late 40s and may last between two and five years in most cases, is called the peri-menopause. During this time a woman's periods become more erratic and gaps between them become longer. Many women begin to have symptoms such as headaches or feelings of irritability or low mood. The 'mid-life crisis' is on its way!

As the peri-menopause nears the actual menopause, other symptoms like hot flushes, night sweats and joint aches and pains may arrive. Levels of the hormones oestrogen and progesterone fall to about 80% of what they were before the peri-menopause began, as egg production ceases and the ovaries become redundant. Finally, the menopause is officially defined as 12 months from the date of your last period, after which naturally occurring pregnancy is no longer possible.

The average age for menopause in the UK is 51, although it can happen much earlier – before 45 it is described as early menopause.

men

The existence of the male menopause (andropause) is a subject of international debate. The pro-andropause theorists claim that around the age of 50 up to 50% of men experience a noticeable or sharp decline in androgen levels (the male sex hormones, which include testosterone) rather than a gentle decline throughout mid and later life, which is the pattern that many endocrinologists perceive in most males.

Symptoms such as decreased sex drive (see pages 178–83), low sperm count, fatigue, night sweats, decline in drive and ambition, and depression have been reported, while the anti-andropause lobby say these symptoms are probably psychological and/or caused by unhealthy living in middle age.

However, even the 'anti' lobby agrees that about 5% of mid-life males do suffer a severe dip in hormonal levels over a short period of time, which can result in loss of libido, muscle and hair, as well as diminished bone density – leaving some men as prone to osteoporosis as post-menopausal women may be.

Whether or not a medical andropause is true for most men – and the issue is far from decided – there is no doubt that many do experience a mid-life physical and emotional crisis.

long-term consequences

While the more debilitating symptoms of the female menopause (described in the panel opposite) are immediately obvious and easy to quantify, in the long-term also, the menopause can have far-reaching effects on health.

While pre-menopausal women have natural protection (via oestrogen) from heart disease, once oestrogen levels drop after the menopause, they are as at risk of heart and circulatory problems as men.

Breast cancer and other cancers also increase significantly in post-menopausal women, while the accelerated bone loss causes a vastly increased risk of developing osteoporosis in later mid life and old age. Many women gain a significant amount of weight during the menopause and in the few years afterwards and, again, medical opinion is divided over whether this is directly related to the hormonal changes – which could slow down the metabolic rate – or is just a lifestyle factor around this age.

Sexual function can be affected, because the loss of oestrogen means that the vaginal wall becomes thinner, less elastic and less moist, while sexual appetite may also be diminished – for a further discussion on these problems, see pages 178–83.

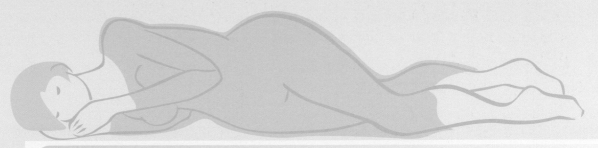

symptoms of the menopause

A woman going through the peri-menopause or menopause may experience some or all of these symptoms – or, occasionally, none at all – which can be sporadic and varying in intensity. Most of these symptoms have also been linked to the male menopause. Strategies for dealing with all these symptoms are discussed on the pages that follow.

hot flushes Often the first sign of the peri-menopause, these can feel like a creeping, claustrophobic heat that may radiate from the chest, face and upper body, lasting for up to several minutes before declining (usually with increased perspiration, especially on face).

night sweats Periods of overheating and profuse sweating during sleep, causing wakefulness and the need to remove bedding to cool the body down.

declining libido Libido may gradually diminish and may be hastened by the discovery that intercourse is painful (see next).

painful intercourse As the vaginal wall changes, and arousal may fail to produce sufficient lubrication, sex may become difficult, which can lead to a decrease in desire in itself.

tiredness Tiredness and lack of energy are often reported, although these may be part of a general decline in physical health that can occur in some women at this age, or because of an over-busy lifestyle.

insomnia Women who have previously slept 'like a log' report that they have trouble getting off to sleep, or wake during the night with their minds racing and can't get back to sleep.

depression Women who have never been prone to depression report unexplained feelings of sadness or misery. Again, some experts believe this isn't a direct medical result of the menopause but a linked reaction to losing fertility and getting older.

irritability and mood swings Many women report a decrease in patience and an increase in irritability and short temper. Well, with so many symptoms to cope with, it is quite understandable... but could have a hormonal base, similar to the depressed mood many women feel before a period. Mood swings are also common.

joint aches and pains Pain or discomfort, tightness and stiffness in the joints, with no arthritis present, are often reported during the menopause and it is thought that these may be linked with hormonal changes altering the make-up of the tissue.

headache or migraine Probably hormonal, as with premenstrual headaches.

poor memory Memory for names, times and appointments seems to be particularly badly affected during the menopause.

coping with the menopause

- Remember that the menopause is not a disease – it is a 'rite of passage'. Say goodbye to your child-bearing years with a tinge of regret but also with a sense of looking forward to the future. Many women in their 50s can testify that a zest for life is psychological, not hormonal, and research shows that a positive attitude to your life can diminish menopausal symptoms. For ideas on improving the quality of your life, see Section 5, Time for Your New Life.

- Freedom from periods and unexpected pregnancy can be a bonus to cherish.

- Much research shows that menopausal symptoms become worse when you are under stress. All the stress-reducing tactics outlined on pages 202–3 may help you to cope without recourse to HRT.

- Smoking, alcohol and caffeine make hot flushes worse, so cut these down or out.

- Reduce the annoyance of hot flushes by taking a hand-held fan plus a small canister of Evian spray water with you in your bag.

- Choose clothes with a low neckline to avoid the claustrophobic feeling that can accompany hot flushes.

- Choose fine-weave clothes in natural fibres – layered in winter – rather than heavy, thick man-made items.

- Acupuncture can help alleviate menopausal symptoms.

- Help prevent osteoporosis by taking 1,500mg a day of calcium citrate.

- Fifteen minutes of weight training a day (see pages 104–7) can strengthen bones as well as muscles.

For females, the standard medical treatment for the past several decades has been with hormone replacement therapy (HRT), which has been claimed to be virtually the elixir of life for women over 50. Medics have promoted it as not only a cure for the worst menopausal symptoms, such as hot flushes and decreased libido, but also as a long-term preventive for heart disease and osteoporosis. Many users claimed to feel reinvigorated and sexy, and to have improved skin, hair and health.

Indeed, HRT using oestrogen and progesterone does seem to work well in eliminating hot flushes and, for as long as it is taken, protect against bone loss (both flushes and bone loss will reoccur if the HRT is stopped). How much of the improvement is due to the 'placebo' effect is, however, a matter of argument – one controlled trial of over 16,000 women published in 2003 concluded that HRT taken over a year did NOT improve well-being and its effects were largely in the mind.

In recent years, however, HRT has caused great controversy in the medical profession. It cannot be taken by women who already have, or have had, breast or womb cancer. For other women, research in the USA and UK shows that the combined oestrogen/progesterone pill can double the risk of breast cancer – and can also increase the risk of heart disease, stroke, blood clots and dementia. Because of these scares – and because around 15% of women experience side-effects like bloating, weight gain, breast tenderness, headaches and nausea when taking HRT – many women have come off it and are keen to try less invasive or more natural alternatives.

other medication

Rather than taking HRT pills, you can use patches, nasal spray or even implants, all of which may be a better alternative for some. Recent research has found that antidepressant drugs known as selective serotonin reuptake inhibitors (SSRIs), such as paroxetine and venlafaxine, can help reduce flushes and night sweats by up to 70% and would, obviously, help depression and anxiety. Raloxifene hydrochloride (brand name Evista) can help prevent osteoporosis and may cut the risk of heart disease and stroke, while bisphosphonate can stop bone loss within six months. See your doctor to discuss the pros and cons of these alternatives in your case.

natural alternatives to HRT

The first line of attack is diet, discussed on pages 54–9. A suitable healthy diet can help avoid weight gain and may reduce other symptoms. Research also shows regular exercise is a good way to minimize hot flushes, as well as to control weight and keep fit. Stretching and yoga can help joint aches and pains, while weight-bearing exercise helps maintain bone density. All types of exercise will help in getting better sleep and promote relaxation and better mood – see Section 2.

supplements and creams

There is a bewildering range of dietary supplements available claiming to control hot flushes and other symptoms. Most haven't been the subject of clinical trials and so their efficacy is mostly anecdotal. There is further information on plant oestrogens and the menopause on pages 56–7. Avoid oestrogenic supplements if you have breast cancer.

Red clover – Contains isoflavones (see page 56 and soya below).

Black cohosh – Routinely used in Germany to treat menopausal symptoms and said to be one of the best relievers for flushes and sweating by acting on the hypothalamus to regulate temperature. It can also ease anxiety, insomnia and mood swings. Currently undergoing large US trials to determine safety and validity. One recent research paper using mice found it could speed the spread of breast cancer, while a clinical trial found it had less effect than a placebo. Nevertheless, it has more professional fans than most of the other herbal remedies.

Dong quai – For hormonal imbalance.

Agnus castus – For hormonal imbalance.

Sage – Said to relieve hot flushes by 56% in a small trial and may help minimize night sweats.

Soya – High in isoflavones, which may give relief from menopausal symptoms and may help to protect bones, though evidence is conflicting. May also help protect against heart disease.

Various supplements mixing two or more of these are widely available. Remember even natural remedies may have hidden dangers or side-effects.

Progesterone creams (like wild yam) are available via the Internet or on prescription (UK), and many women find 2–3ml rubbed into fatty areas of the skin helps reduce hot flushes, but their effectiveness against osteoporosis or cancer isn't clinically proven.

tips for the male menopause

In most males, androgens (hormones such as testosterone) drop at around 1% per annum after the 30s, rather than there being an 80% drop within a few short years, as is the case with the female menopause. However, about 5% of men suffer androgen deficiency syndrome, when the male hormone replacement therapy (TRT) may be useful.

There is evidence that implants are more effective than testosterone pills, which, for men experiencing the normal gradual drop in hormones, have not proved effective in improving sexual function. For erection problems, Viagra is a better bet for most. For more information on improving libido in mid life, see Libido on pages 178–83. Testosterone has not been shown to improve bone density in men.

Whether the decline in androgen levels is sharp or more gradual, a number of men report hot flushes during mid life. There is a definite link – when men suffering from prostate cancer have androgen deprivation as part of their therapy, 80% suffer from hot flushes and sleep disturbance.

Factors which may speed the reduction of testosterone levels in men include stress, weight gain, high alcohol intake and lack of exercise. So the moral seems to be – lead a healthy life with plenty of activity and relaxation.

- Avoid a BMI over 27 or 28.

- Slow down your pace of work to match your energy levels.

- Take daily regular aerobic (e.g. walking) and weight-bearing (e.g. weights) exercise.

- Have no more than 2 glasses of alcohol a day and take 2 days off from drinking a week.

- Enjoy life.

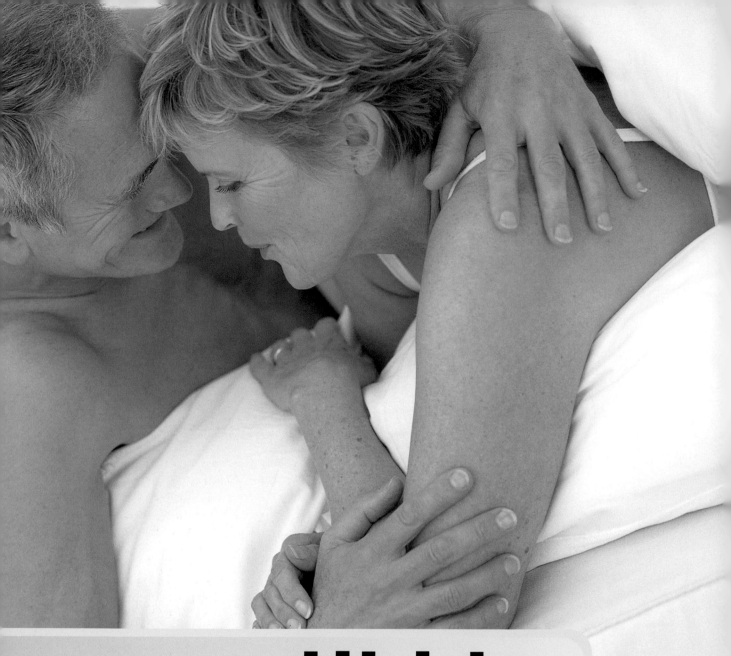

well-being and libido

There really is no standard for libido. It is totally subjective and so all that matters is that you – and your partner – are happy with what you have. One thing is for certain – you don't have to have sex to make love. Here we consider the difference between sex and lovemaking, and look at all the ways that libido can be boosted – if you feel that's what you need.

The first thing you should know about libido is that the statistics you read in the papers and magazines about how often other people have sex rarely paint an accurate picture. The fact is that more people lie about sex than about any other human function. Everyone wants others to think they have sex more often than they do.

lies, damn lies and statistics

So any statistician hoping to get the truth is wasting his or her time. For example, a recent study in the USA from the National Opinion Research Center at Chicago University, investigating sexual habits in people over 50, found there was only a marginal decline in the amount of sexual activity (5 times a month) compared with young adults (6–7 times a month). In another study, 90% of men aged 80 or over said they were still sexually active. This may, of course, all be accurate – but it may not. The clinical fact is that the physical sex drive declines with age because, in mid-life and old age, levels of the sex hormones decline.

does declining libido matter?

When it comes to sex, the only thing that really matters is whether or not you are happy with your situation. There is evidence that a reasonably high percentage of long- (and presumably fairly happily) married couples in mid life don't have sex at all, and are perfectly satisfied with that. Other single people (perhaps divorced or widowed) give up sex and are happy to remain celibate. Problems only arise when one or other partner is unhappy with their sex life, or when a single or newly divorced person finds they can't get an erection, or can't face sex with someone even if attracted to them. Seek help from a doctor if you think you or your partner may have a medical problem that is affecting your sex life. Many problems can be easily resolved.

Even if you can't have intercourse every night – or every month – what you CAN do is make love. Kissing, cuddling and snuggling up together – are all as important – or more important – than actual sex.

the trouble with sex ...

If you are unhappy with the quality of your own libido, that of your partner, or your sex life in general, there is plenty that can be done to improve matters. We look at the most common reasons why your sex life can take a downturn in mid life, and discuss how you might deal with them ...

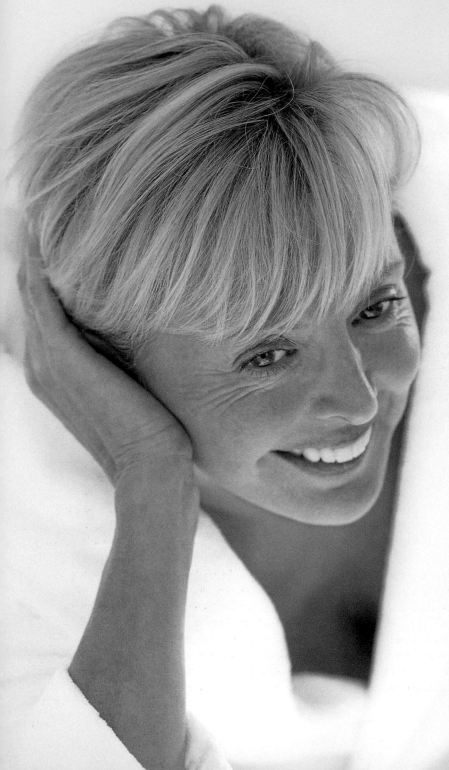

the natural decline of sex hormones

As we saw in the last chapter on the menopause and andropause, mid life is a time when the sexual hormone levels can drop rapidly – certainly for women, while for many men, it is a more gentle decline, the cumulative effect of which becomes noticeable around fifty. A drop in these hormones is a major reason for a lessening of desire in both sexes and what is sometimes coyly termed a 'decline in sexual performance' in men.

Conventional hormone replacement therapy can improve libido in women, while TRT (male HRT, using testosterone) can have a similar effect for men, and new research says testosterone can also be used to enhance enjoyment of sex by women.

All hormonal treatments are available in pill, patch, injection, implant and other forms – see your doctor for advice. However, not everyone wants to try drug therapy, and for many people a decline in the regularity or urgency of sex may be something they find acceptable ... it is the body telling us that our child-bearing years are coming to a natural end. That said, one recent report finds that 50% of males aged 70 are still fully potent (i.e. able to get and maintain erection and achieve ejaculation) and for many women, having a man take longer is actually a bonus. For both sexes, greater attention to foreplay and 'taking your time' can more than make up for any shortfalls in hormones.

the natural ageing process
Several factors have a bearing on sexual function as we age. In men, nerve impulses slow down, which decreases genital sensitivity, and the arteries in the penis are less able to maintain the blood pressure necessary for an erection, which may cause erectile dysfunction (see also Poor health, Psychological factors and Lifestyle opposite and page 182). Viagra and the new rash of similar drugs are designed to overcome erectile problems by increasing blood flow to the penis, and these are the best solution for most older men. Other variations on the theme are coming along too – there are creams that claim to work more quickly than sidenafil (Viagra's active agent). Ask your doctor for advice. Non-chemical ways to improve potency include the natural herbs gingko biloba, ginseng and tribulus terrestrus.

For women, vaginal lubrication may be a problem and, as in men, a decline in blood circulation may mean less sensitivity in the area. The walls of the vagina also become thinner and less elastic and this can make sexual intercourse difficult and may cause tearing of the vaginal lining and/or pain. A doctor can prescribe jelly for simple lubrication, or oestrogen-containing creams. There is also a device approved by the US Food and Drug Administration called the Eros CTD, a vacuum instrument that improves blood flow to the vaginal area.

Herbs that may help females include dong quai, said to improve vaginal lubrication, aloe vera juice, and damiana, said to increase sex drive, while vitamins C and E can help maintain vaginal tissue.

For both sexes, 'use it or lose it' is a good maxim – research shows regular sex, three times a week

for preference – does keep the sexual organs working better, no matter your age, with foreplay of extreme importance for both sexes. Daily pelvic floor squeezing for women also helps maintain muscle tone in the vaginal area, while aerobic exercise improves circulation (including to the penis) for men.

poor health
Research has found, hardly surprisingly, that in mid and old age it is those who retain good health who are most likely to continue with an active sex life, while people in poor health are most likely to be celibate. Diabetes and athero-sclerosis (hardening of the arteries) are both known to have an effect on erectile function in men. (See also Drugs, Lifestyle and Psychological factors).

Likewise, a good sex life improves your health. Sex improves the circulation, can lower blood levels of 'bad' cholesterol, cause relaxation hormones to be released and thus relieve stress, release natural pain-killing endorphins and keep the prostate healthy.

drugs
It is estimated that 25% of all male impotence is induced by prescription or over-the-counter drugs. Known culprits include some types of medication for high blood pressure, non-steroidal anti-inflammatory drugs, tranquillizers, antihistamines and many antidepressants (although depression itself can cause impotence – see Psychological Factors – so these latter statistics may be suspect). Recreational drugs, like cannabis, can also reduce libido, as can alcohol and tobacco (see Lifestyle).

psychological factors
Stress, anxiety, fatigue and, most of all, depression can contribute to libido loss in both sexes and impotence in men. About 90% of depressed men suffer some degree of impotence. The answer is to treat these psychological causes – which can be nothing to do with sex, but are often related to problems at work or in other areas of home and family life.

lifestyle A well-balanced lifestyle can boost sexual performance and libido. At least in part, this means leading a healthy day-to-day life, with moderation in most things the key. Keep alcohol intake low (even fairly moderate amounts of alcohol can cause 'brewer's droop' at any age, and can dull the nerves to the female sex organs too). Nicotine too can anaesthetize the sex organs. Lack of regular exercise appears to be directly linked to poor sexual function, and you need to do not only aerobic exercise to increase circulation, but also loosening and stretching exercises, particularly of the neck and shoulders. Tight neck muscles can restrict the circulation around the head and neck and may impede the work of the hypothalamus, which regulates all hormonal functions.

A good diet is very important. Several of the foods in The Top 20 Foods for Anti-ageing on pages 20-3 have a good effect on your libido – particularly those high in antioxidants, and a generally healthy diet will boost health (see Poor health). The classic libidinous foods, oysters, are rich in zinc, but if you don't happen to like them, plenty of nuts, seeds, whole grains, other seafood and leafy greens – all good sources of the mineral – will do the trick.

emotional baggage Even if your hormones are still raging, you both look great and you still want sex, sometimes years of built-up negative emotions directed at your partner can dull libido so much that you just can't do it with that person any more. Women seem more prone to sexual turn-off because of psychological factors, but they can easily affect men too. Research shows that anger is the emotion most likely to diminish desire for your partner – resentment, frustration, fear, unspoken issues. If the cause(s) of these feelings can be resolved, sex life can often be restored too. Counselling together may be an idea.

the question of familiarity There has been recent debate on the fact that lessening desire for the same person over time is quite normal and natural. When someone is new and exciting, sex is also new and exciting. If, though, you've lived with someone for twenty, thirty or forty years – and know every inch of their anatomy and their habits – excitement hardly comes into it. If you feel you or your partner may simply be feeling bored with sex, the most tried and tested methods of getting that frisson back is either to use what are now termed 'sex toys' (widely available in sex shops or on the Internet) or to try sex videos/manuals, or any other erotica, to get aroused together.

Of course, perhaps your partner is no longer attracted to you. Blunt as this sounds, you might not be getting sex from your partner because he or she just doesn't fancy the way you look any more. Visual appeal is a huge part of sexual attraction for most of us. Not just for sex appeal but also for our well-being and confidence, it is important not to 'let yourself go'. Other sections of this book aim to help you stay looking really good (Exercise, Looks) – and not just 'for your age' but really good, full stop. If it is you who no longer fancies your partner, then encouragement for them to scrub up and shape up is called for.

the reproductive years are over The main point of sex is to procreate the human race. Whoever invented it made it so good when we are young because that is when we are fertile. Obviously there are women and men in their mid life who still have children – and men can be fertile into their 80s – but once the reproductive years are at an end the original motivation for sex may no longer be there. Although few people admit it, for a lot of women in particular, sex is more about having babies than about pleasure. There are, no doubt, many thousands of men in their 40s and 50s wondering why their wives no longer want sex and this may be the simple answer. This is something that needs discussing, not ignoring.

simple ways to boost your libido

- **don't worry about what you think others do** Just think about what you (and your partner) want to do. Your sex life is not a competition. Massage each other or just cuddle – sex may follow naturally if you stop worrying.

- **talk to your partner** Not everyone can feel like sex all the time. Keep up good communication so you can explain, without loss of face or rancour on their part, when you feel like it and when you don't. Expect the same of them. Knowing you can both do this makes sex very much better when you do do it.

- **enjoy life** Research shows that people who lead an interesting life, have fun and regularly circulate with new people find their sex lives improve.

- **use it so you don't lose it** Research shows that people who have sex regularly find it easier and more pleasurable than those who only have it occasionally. Even if at first you find it a bit of a 'chore', libido DOES return the more often you have sex, and for women, vaginal lubrication improves too.

- **keep an open mind** Many people give up on sex because they feel it isn't 'normal' to want it as they get older. A positive attitude can work wonders.

- **look at the positives of changing sexual performance or appetite** For example, as men get older they may not be able to have an orgasm six times a night, but they can 'keep going for longer' each time they do have sex.

- **a new relationship** – or reworking the boundaries of an old one – can reawaken libido. Time apart from a long-term partner may do the trick.

- **get something new into your sex life** While I abhor advice to women to wear frilly pants around the house and dress up in silk stockings and little else to greet your partner as he arrives home (it's more likely to embarrass or frighten the guy), a bit of sexual titillation is always a good idea... sexy underwear in the bedroom, a sex manual, a soft-porn DVD ... that kind of thing.

- **people in good health enjoy sex more** Eat well, exercise regularly, and avoid too much alcohol, cigarettes or recreational drugs, all of which affect libido and sexual functioning.

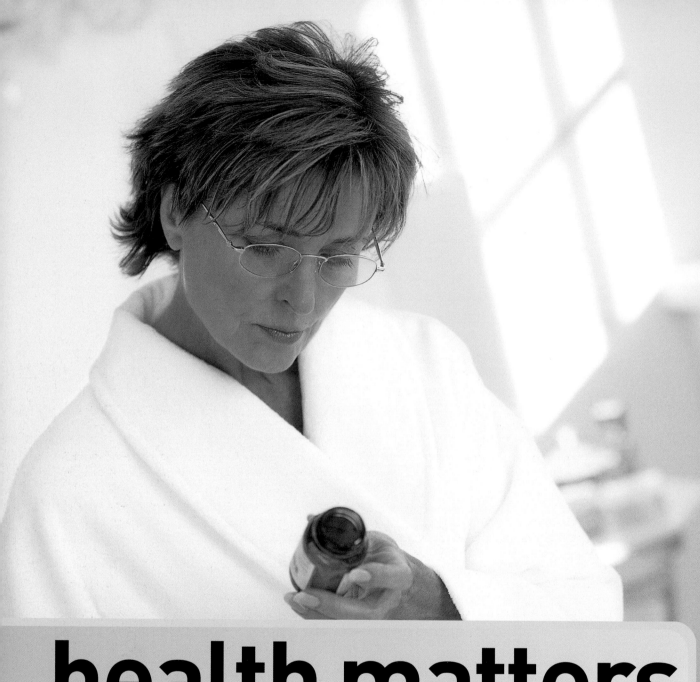

health matters

In order to enjoy your life you need a certain standard of health – in other words, the best health you can have given your circumstances and what has gone before. This chapter aims to help you deal with the most common health problems of mid life.

As you read through this chapter you may feel that you suffer from more than your fair share of the complaints and illnesses that it describes. Even if you have not felt that you were in blooming good health in recent years, it is surprising what can be achieved with even minimal attention to yourself and/or lifestyle changes.

If you are in good shape, however, it is still important to take care of yourself as a preventive measure … for good health is even more vital as you get older. It is your key to independence and the single most wished-for factor when people are asked what they want for their old age.

We will look at the most common syndrome associated with mid life, 'tired all the time', and the associated complaints of lethargy and lack of energy. These syndromes may have both physical and psychological causes, all of which we discuss.

Of course, if you are tired, you may have insomnia. Nearly everyone in mid life suffers from this at least some of the time and, in the long term, it can have a drastic effect on your life and that of those close to you. The tips that I give are those that have worked best for others.

The second most common group of complaints in mid life is 'aches and pains' – whether from arthritis or other muscular-skeletal problems. If you are forced to spend much of the day being painfully aware of your body, this dominates everything. There is, however, much you can do to improve the situation.

It is said that 65% of over-40s have what they consider to be a poor digestive system, complaining most frequently of (in descending order) heartburn, bloating, irritable bowel and constipation … We look at what can be done, and discuss the relevance of overindulgence in alcohol, tobacco and recreational drugs.

Two-thirds of us will eventually get some form of cancer or heart disease … we examine how you can help beat the odds and keep at bay these potential killers – as well as the other big disease of middle age, diabetes.

Lastly, a healthy body needs a healthy mind, so if anxiety, stress, depression or poor memory drag you down, even if only occasionally, we have some solutions with which to end the chapter.

tiredness and lethargy If you are physically and mentally shattered or lacking in energy for much of your day, the problem needs resolving – 'tired all the time' is a growing problem and, for many, it first occurs in mid life.

the many causes of tiredness

Trying to pinpoint exactly what is causing your feelings of tiredness may not be simple, as there are many possible explanations. Here are the main potential causes.

Being female! Women are more prone to tiredness than men, according to a Scottish study (by men!) published in the *British Medical Journal*. This is thought to be because women are more conditioned to do multi-tasking, rather than because they are in any way the 'weaker sex'. So if you are female, try to make a special effort to pace yourself, don't ignore the need for a rest now and then, and get enough sleep. If you have PMS or are in the menopause, you are even more likely to feel tired as, due to hormonal changes, fatigue is a common complaint at both these times. Good diet and enough exercise will help.

Depression People with a history of depression are much more likely to report feeling tired. So if you think your tiredness may have psychological origins, see your doctor and/or a therapist for help, and see also Mind Matters (page 198). If your depression is 'circumstantial' – i.e. there are factors in your life that are bringing you down, then Section 5 may help.

Emotional stress Even if you aren't depressed, emotional strain can bring you down, especially in the long term. Permanent overwork, too many things to juggle, relationship problems, family troubles … All these can increase tiredness. Relaxation techniques and a conscious effort to build time for yourself are important.

Physical stress When your body is under stress it is normal for it to react by feeling tired. Stress of the kind that makes you have symptoms of nervousness or anxiety (palpitations, dry mouth, perspiration, for example) causes the release of adrenaline and if this is prolonged it will literally wear you out. Get regular daily exercise to help release this adrenaline, and see pages 202–3 for dealing with stress.

Medical conditions Illness is another stress for the body – coping with serious illness in the short term (e.g. a bad bout of 'flu) or in the long term can make you tired – you need to make sure to give yourself time to 'be ill' and time to recover. Several medical conditions are recognized as having tiredness as one of their symptoms. These include Epstein Barr (glandular fever), 'flu and bronchitis, anaemia, cancer, diabetes, hypothyroidism, multiple sclerosis, liver disease, heart and lung disease. They also include disorders such as sleep apnoea and chronic fatigue syndrome. See your doctor if you feel a medical condition could be causing your tiredness.

Lack of rest Obvious as it sounds, one common cause of tiredness and lack of energy is 'overdoing it'. If you are on the go all day every day, you are going to feel tired some of the time. It isn't always necessary to be busy sixteen hours a day (see Section 5).

Too much rest Ah! But too much rest can also make you feel tired – probably by reducing the amount of oxygen that gets to the brain. For more on this, see pages 188–90.

Poor quality of sleep Even if you get 7 or 8 hours in bed, you may be tired because you have poor sleep patterns or even sleep apnoea. See overleaf.

Poor exercise and lifestyle habits Too little exercise can make you feel tired and reduce your body's capacity to deal with a busy life. Exercise is one of the best 'cures' for daytime tiredness and lack of energy, as long as it is moderate (e.g. walking) rather than hard/vigorous. In the short term, the increase in blood circulation – and, therefore, available oxygen – has a regenerating effect on the brain, which is the seat of much fatigue. In the long term, increased fitness can help you keep going for longer.

Poor diet Can induce tiredness by not providing enough of the energy-converting vitamins and other nutrients. Drastic dieting can also mean that there aren't enough calories available to provide energy.

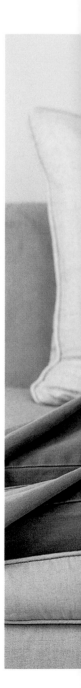

8

ideas for boosting energy levels and banishing tiredness

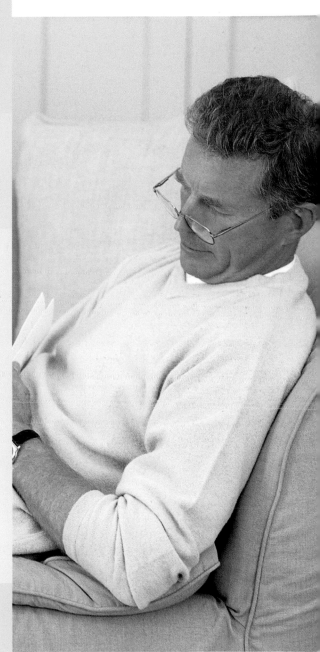

- **eat a balanced breakfast** to sustain you through the morning and have a high-protein lunch containing only small amounts of good-quality carbs. A lunch high in carbs, especially those such as white bread or white pasta, will make you feel tired in the afternoon as they encourage production of sleep-inducing hormones.

- **get as much fresh air as you can** Try to work in a room where you can have the window open; and sleep with the window ajar. Stale air makes you feel stagnant.

- **keep the heat down low** If your brain is too warm, you will soon feel tired and your brain will slow down.

- **avoid sugary drinks and snacks** for energy during the day. The boost they give will be short-term, and within an hour you'll feel more tired than ever. Instead have small amounts of lean protein, like yoghurt or nuts and seeds.

- **for an instant reviver**, do 1 minute's skipping or marching on the spot, with arms moving, or running up and down stairs. This increases circulation and carries oxygen to the brain.

- **take a 5-minute siesta** Research shows that this fits in with the body's circadian rhythms and people who take a nap, say, mid-afternoon, perform better for the rest of the day than people who don't.

- **several supplements** are claimed to help improve energy levels. Co-enzyme Q10 is particularly good for improving stamina for exercise. Acetyl-l-carnitine and alpha lipoic acid used together may increase energy by boosting mitochondria, the internal combustion engine of cells. Iron pills may help, even if you are not anaemic.

- **drink 2 litres of fluids a day** – preferably water. Your brain needs to be only 3% dehydrated to affect mental and physical performance considerably.

insomnia and sleep
Research shows that 52% of us would choose a good night's sleep over sex or a pay rise, and that two-thirds of us have trouble sleeping at some time during our lives – often, this occurs in the middle decades.

Sleep deprivation can, in the short term, make you less productive at work, irritable, less able to concentrate, less able to learn, and may even make you feel confused. In the longer term, it can cause anxiety, depression, loss of libido and impaired tissue repair, and can blunt the immune system.

Researchers are not all agreed on how much sleep is necessary for good health but the majority seem to favour 7–8 hours a night – and women appear to need slightly more sleep than men (about half an hour). During this time, we need a good balance of slow-wave, or delta, sleep (the deepest, body-restorative sleep when human growth hormone is at its most active) and REM sleep (dreaming sleep, which, it is thought, is vital for a healthy brain). These types of sleep go in cycles through the night, with longer periods of REM towards the end of the sleeping period.

what causes insomnia?
It often begins with a period of emotional stress and/or depression, (e.g. job loss, bereavement) when insomnia is usual and normal, but the wakeful pattern can easily become established and then a habit. As the sufferer becomes increasingly anxious about the lack of sleep, this creates a vicious circle, with worries about not sleeping beginning during the evening.

For entrenched insomnia of this type, cognitive behaviour therapy (CBT) works well for most, while for milder cases a relaxing evening routine and self-help tactics can do the trick, although this can take time.

Sometimes insomnia can be caused by lifestyle. High alcohol intake is associated with middle-of-the-night waking – alcohol disturbs the brain chemicals that promote the deep-sleep phase and also promotes fluctuations in blood sugar levels which can produce low blood sugar around 3am. It can also contribute to sleep apnoea (opposite). Drinking too much of any liquid in the evening can cause you to wake to go to the toilet (and, as we get older, our bladders do become less able to hold in quantity).

It is hard for the brain to relax into sleep if you work late – try to stop work at least three hours before you go to bed. Shift work and jet lag are known to disrupt sleep patterns. Caffeine intake should be stopped by mid-afternoon at the latest,

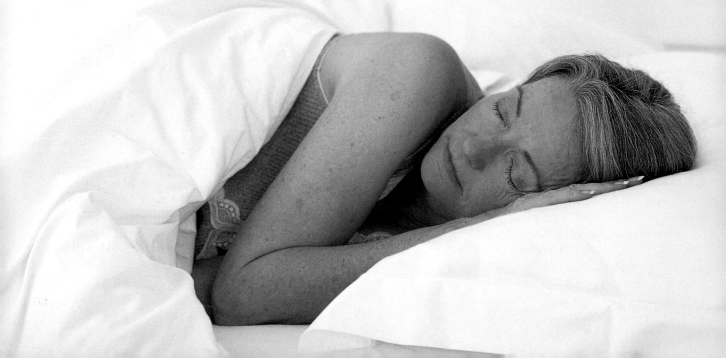

as caffeine induces wakefulness. Some drugs can cause insomnia – e.g. certain antidepressants, some asthma drugs (e.g. prednisolone) and heart medication such as digoxin. Vigorous exercise too soon before bed can keep you awake by stimulating the production of adrenaline … but sex is good, as it releases calming hormones. Foods rich in tyramine (a compound linked to wakefulness) can affect sleep and dream patterns, so avoid overripe cheeses, red wine and pickles in the evening. Eating too late can give you night-time indigestion or heartburn, which can keep you awake; however, too little to eat in the evening can keep you awake with hunger pangs.

so what can be done?

Apart from the relaxing tips in the box on the right or, for chronic insomnia, cognitive behaviour therapy (CBT), certain foods, drinks and herbs are known to help promote good sleep:

Foods rich in tryptophan, an amino acid which converts into calming serotonin in the brain – one of the endorphins, neurotransmitters that are the body's 'feel-good' drugs. Turkey, bananas, milk, nuts and dried apricots all contain high levels.

Starchy carbohydrates, such as whole-grain cereals: these also increase production of serotonin. Make sure your evening meal includes some good-quality starch (e.g. whole-wheat pasta, brown rice, whole-grain bread) and just before bed have a small snack that includes both tryptophan and serotonin – such as a banana sandwich.

Foods rich in vitamin B6 This vitamin promotes serotonin levels in the brain – oats are a good source, as are other whole grains, turkey and walnuts.

Foods rich in magnesium and calcium Both of these minerals help induce calmness. Milk is an excellent calcium source, while nuts, seeds, pulses and green veg are good for magnesium. Lettuce contains lactucarium, which is a natural sedative.

Herbs and herbal supplements can be almost as good as a prescription sleeping pill – some of the best are valerian, passiflora, camomile and lemon balm. There is also a supplement called 5-HTP which is said to help tryptophan convert into serotonin.

Prescription sleeping pills should be used only rarely or for short periods (e.g. during a high-stress situation like bereavement). Constant use increases tolerance, so you need more and more for the same effect. These pills also alter your sleep patterns.

tips for a good night's sleep

- To get into a regular routine that prepares your mind to realize that you'll be sleeping soon, incorporate some or all of the following tips.

- An hour or two before bed, do some gentle exercise, such as a walk around the garden or a short walk with the dog, or 15 minutes of yoga or stretching. Exercise helps release endorphins.

- Do nothing that taxes the brain in the evening. Ideal occupations are watching a light comedy on TV, listening to a play on the radio or reading a popular novel. You want to induce a state of happiness and calm.

- Avoid arguments/heated discussion in the evening.

- Take a warm bath using calming herbal essences such as camomile or lavender.

- Dim the lights an hour before bedtime in whatever room you are and make sure your bedroom lights can be switched to dim too.

- Have your sleep-inducing snack/drink after your bath, just before you clean your teeth and go to bed.

- Snorers disturb their own sleep as well as others. Alcohol and smoking make it worse, and large evening meals make it more likely. So lose weight, and avoid drinking, smoking and late eating. Sleep on your side and try to breathe through your nose not your mouth. Anti-snoring devices (clips, sprays, etc.) have mixed success.

sleep apnoea

Obstructive sleep apnoea (OSA), affecting up to 8% of snorers (mostly overweight middle-aged males), can be life-threatening. In OSA, the breathing stops altogether for short periods up to 300 times a night, causing the sufferer to wake fighting for breath. See your doctor if you suspect you are affected (chronic fatigue and morning headaches are the usual symptoms).

aches and pains Joint, muscular and other aches and pains
can cause much misery in mid life, but there is plenty you can do to ease these problems.

arthritis

The word 'arthritis' means damage to, or disease of, the joints. There two most common types are osteo-arthritis, affecting over 1 million people in the UK, and rheumatoid arthritis, affecting about 350,000.

Osteoarthritis affects about 80% people over 50 to some degree and is sometimes called 'wear and tear', because the cartilage cushioning the joints thins and may wear out completely. This causes pain, stiffness and sometimes swelling, as well as other changes in the joint, and can limit range of movement. It's common in the knees, hips, hands and spine, and is not usually associated with redness and heat in the area.

Obesity can put extra strain on the lower joints and make arthritis worse. While medical treatment is usually confined to painkillers or non-steroidal anti-inflammatory drugs (NSAIDs) – and sometimes, eventually, joint replacement – there is much you can do to help minimize the negative side-effects of arthritis (see the panel opposite).

Rheumatoid arthritis is an inflammatory disease occurring more often in women than in men, and more frequently in younger adults than osteoarthritis, often beginning with weakness and pain in the hands. Although there is a theory that an infection may be the cause, this hasn't been proved. The disease can be unpredictable, with periods of remission, but eventually joints may become swollen, red and inflamed. Other symptoms can include tiredness, loss of weight, feeling unwell, fever and night sweats, and even a rash or mouth ulcers. Many of the helpful hints for osteoarthritis are also useful (see opposite).

fibromyalgia

This painful condition of the muscles, tendons and/or ligaments, rather than in the joints, tends to hit around the late 40s, and only one in ten sufferers is male. There may be multiple sore points around the body – often in the shoulders, outer elbows or chest.

Sufferers often sleep badly and, vice versa, may develop fibromyalgia if they have chronic insomnia. The condition is also linked with depression, stress and trauma, and there is no diagnostic test as it is a descriptive term rather than a medical condition. Fibromyalgia can spontaneously get better, and can sometimes be improved with regular moderate exercise. The good news is sufferers are not at higher risk of arthritis. See opposite for further tips.

polymyalgia rheumatica (PMR)

This is a disease which can be diagnosed by a blood test and tends to affect around four in every thousand people over 50. The cause is unknown, but symptoms are pain and stiffness (worse in the mornings) often around the shoulders and thighs, and perhaps feeling unwell and tired. There may also be inflammation in the arteries around the temple in severe cases. Treatment is usually steroids, which may be needed for several years – the condition can often be cured but may be almost permanent in some. All the other aches and pains described above can be mistaken for PMR, so diagnosis is important.

headaches

There are very many possible causes of headache, including hormonal changes, stress, dehydration, diet, illness (e.g. infection or fever). Most headaches are short-lived and can be controlled with over-the-counter painkillers – but don't rely on these, as research shows that they can actually, with overuse, make headaches worse. Migraine headaches can often be improved with feverfew tincture or tablets. If prone to frequent unexplained headaches it would be a good idea to see your doctor for a check-up.

other aches and pains

'Rheumatism' is a blanket expression for unexplained aches and pains around the joints. Tennis elbow and housemaid's knee are examples of rheumatism.

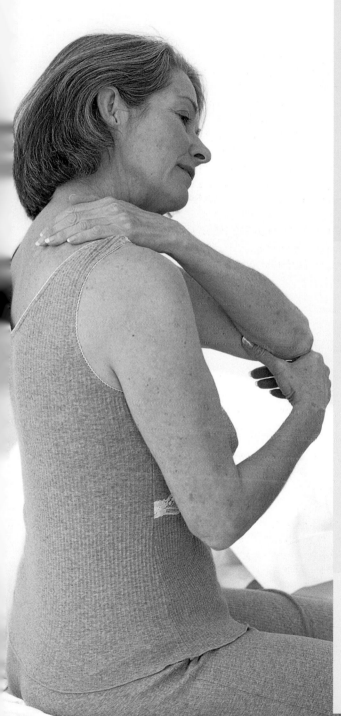

beating arthritis and other aches and pains

Use the tips that are most appropriate to your case –
and see your doctor for further advice.

- **special diet** Many words have been written about
special exclusion diets to help arthritis, but the UK
Arthritis Research Campaign says that, other than
maintaining a healthy weight and eating a balanced diet,
there is rarely any benefit in eating a special diet, and that
an unusual diet may do more harm than good. They say,
'Occasionally, someone with arthritis finds that a specific
type of food upsets them but this is unusual.' Foods most
often claimed to make arthritis worse are citrus fruits,
potatoes, tomatoes, aubergines and peppers, coffee and
red wine. Meat may also be a trigger for rheumatoid
arthritis, one 2000 study found – and recent research
published in late 2003 shows that meat contains a type of
molecule which the tissues can absorb and which may
cause inflammation.

- **the omega-3 oils in oily fish** and cod liver
oil have been proved to be helpful in relieving the pain
and disability of arthritis. If you don't enjoy oily fish, take
fish oil supplements instead – 1000mg a day is normal.

- **keep your body weight down** – vital for
helping osteoarthritis.

- **several supplements** may help the pain and
stiffness of arthritis and other muscular-skeletal
complaints. These include bromelian, an enzyme found
in pineapples, the spices ginger and turmeric, glucosamine
(which can help form joint cartilage), chondroitin (which
works well together with glucosamine to keep the joints
healthy) and methyl sulphonyl methane (MSM), which
is another component of cartilage structure. Collagen
supplements may stimulate the growth of new cartilage
and help pain, while the herbs nettles, rue and boswellian
are said to be anti-inflammatory. Green-lipped mussels
and devil's claw may also work for some. For tight muscles
and stiffness, the mineral magnesium can act as a relaxer.

- **regular gentle-to-moderate exercise**
works to maintain joint mobility – yoga, stretching and
swimming are all ideal. All joints should be put through
their full range of movement once a day, to prevent
stiffening up.

- **a heat pad** placed on the site of pain can help, as
can a cold pad.

the digestive system
When we are young, the digestive system can often take a great deal of abuse or be ignored and still behave in an impeccable manner. As we get older, however, this is no longer the case. The gut needs a lot of looking after! So, starting from the top …

heartburn/indigestion

Heartburn – pain behind the breastbone, often radiating to neck and arm, caused by stomach acids rising into the gullet – is frequently mistaken for a heart attack, while dyspepsia or indigestion refers to general pain and discomfort in the abdominal area and chest.

Heartburn is most frequently caused by overweight, eating large meals, bending over, or smoking. Younger women find it common during pregnancy. Frequent heartburn can be a sign of hiatus hernia and you should get it checked by your doctor.

Dyspepsia can be caused by irritation of the stomach lining and/or duodenum, which may be due to overeating, anxiety, or certain foods/drinks – fatty foods, spices, coffee and alcohol are the most common. Some drugs can also irritate the stomach and cause ulcers, notably aspirin and some NSAIDs (non-steroidal anti-inflammatory drugs).

CURES: Over-the-counter antacid remedies may work, but shouldn't be relied on too much. Best advice? Stop smoking, maintain a suitable weight, eat small frequent meals, avoid foods/drinks you know trigger attacks, and see your doctor to check if other problems (e.g. peptic ulcer) could be the cause.

bloating

The most common cause of bloating is a meal rich in carbohydrates, particularly refined white carbs based on grains – white bread, white pasta, cakes or biscuits. Carbs act like blotting paper to retain liquid in the body. A high-salt snack or meal has a similar effect – the body retains fluid to try to dilute the salt to a reasonable level, as high sodium concentrations can be dangerous. Thirdly, intestinal wind (gas) can cause bloating – typical causes of a gassy stomach are pulses (beans, chickpeas, lentils), onions, cabbage and other brassicas, wheat and dried fruits. All these foods are 'good for you', so rather than eliminating them, eat them well cooked, finely chopped or puréed, in small amounts. Women

pre-period or during the menopause may be more prone to bloating – fresh fruits, salads and lean protein should not produce this effect. In general, chew food thoroughly, eat little and often, and try to relax while eating … stressful meals can cause bloating.

irritable bowel syndrome

Between 12 and 20% of the UK population – and twice as many women as men – suffer from IBS, which is not so much a disease as a set of symptoms that may vary from person to person, and may come and go. The most common are abdominal cramps and pain, bloating, flatulence, and either loose bowels or constipation, perhaps alternating.

There are links between the onset of IBS and stress, and it may be triggered by illness, or can be caused by food intolerance. Wheat and dairy products are the two most common allergens for IBS sufferers and indeed the symptoms are similar to those of lactose intolerance (inability to digest the sugars in milk products). A course of probiotics (available from pharmacies and health food shops – only buy if kept in the fridge) may also help relieve IBS by colonizing the gut with gut-friendly bacteria.

Relaxation and cognitive behaviour therapy seem to improve symptoms by up to 70%, while a basic elimination diet can find out if you are intolerant of any food(s). In general, a healthy diet and lifestyle including regular exercise may help.

constipation

One in six people – most often women – suffer from constipation, and many of these are aged over 50. Usually the problem can be fairly easily overcome with correct diet and exercise (see 10 Ways to Keep Regular opposite) and this is the most sensible way to treat it rather than resorting to laxatives, which can upset the natural balance of the intestines and bowel. The body can also become used to them, so that you need more and more for them to work.

10 ways to keep regular

- **include high-fibre foods** at every meal, with a balance of both soluble and insoluble fibre.

- **find insoluble fibre in** whole-grain bread, cereals, brown rice and wholewheat pasta; in leafy green vegetables, nuts and seeds; and in reasonable quantities in other vegetables, fruit and pulses.

- **find soluble fibre in** most fresh and dried fruits, especially citrus fruits, apples, mangoes; in pulses; and also in reasonable quantities in oats, barley and rye.

- **aim for at least 6g of total fibre per meal** – most food packaging carry fibre information. If already constipated, aim for 8g fibre per meal.

- **eat 7 portions of fruit and vegetables a day**, and eat whole fruit rather than fruit juice, which has the fibre removed.

- **drink 2 litres of liquids a day** and aim for at least half of this to be water. Without enough liquid, high-fibre foods cannot do their job of increasing the bulk of stools and making them pass easily through the gut.

- **prunes and rhubarb** contain compounds that help ease constipation, so can be included in your diet a few times a week.

- **go for natural 'health food' remedies** rather than harsh laxatives from the chemist. Rosehip syrup, olive oil, honey, liquorice, molasses, psyllium seeds and curry spices all have a laxative effect.

- **a course of probiotics will also help** – these are natural gut bacteria which for most people seem to have a laxative effect.

- **take regular daily exercise** – both aerobic exercise, such as brisk walking, and other exercise, such as toning or weight training, will help stimulate the gut into action.

the big three
Heart disease, cancer and diabetes are the three diseases most likely to affect people in mid life. Here we look at the implications...

heart disease

CVD (cardiovascular disease – disease of the heart and/or blood vessels) accounts for 235,000 deaths a year in the UK, with coronary heart disease (CHD) claiming 125,000 of these. There are annually 270,000 heart attacks and 93,000 middle-aged men are diagnosed with heart disease. However, women are by no means immune – they are now at almost as high a risk of CVD as men, and four times as many women die from it as from breast cancer. CVD is most likely to hit men over 45 and women over 55 – and the major risk factors, other than genetics, stem from your choice of lifestyle.

A diet for a healthy heart needs to be low in saturated fat – recent research shows that even an excess 100g of saturates a week can increase women's risk of dying from heart disease by nearly 38%. Monounsaturated fats (e.g. olive oil) and omega-3 fats (e.g. from oily fish) can, on the other hand, protect the heart. Leafy vegetables (rich in B vitamins B6, B12 and folic acid to help prevent high homocysteine levels in the blood, which can be a significant factor in CVD), all fruit and vegetables, nuts, garlic, pulses, soya and red wine, and the plant chemicals they contain, are all linked with a healthy heart (see Section 1).

Lack of exercise is another major factor. The British Heart Foundation recommends half an hour of moderate aerobic exercise five times a week. but research shows that almost any exercise is better than none – e.g. 10 minutes a day or 20 minutes three times a week. See Section 2 for more information.

Good diet and exercise will help prevent overweight or obesity, which are high risk factors, and they will also help prevent high blood pressure and a poor blood-fats profile (high in LDL cholesterol, homocysteine and triglycerides), which are both risk factors for CVD.

A high percentage of heart deaths are due to tobacco smoking (which increases the blood's capacity to clot) and drugs such as cocaine can also cause heart failure. Alcohol is fine for most people in small amounts (1–2 glasses a day have a beneficial effect on the heart for people in mid life and later), but heavy and binge drinking are linked with heart attacks.

Stress can also cause CVD – a study of over 3,000 adults showed a definite link between long-term anger, anxiety, impatience and stress with increased blood pressure and, therefore, heart disease. Overwork really can kill – working 60 hours a week doubles the risk of a coronary. On the other hand, getting enough sleep and laughter, and anti-stress devices, like stroking pets, can reduce blood pressure and dangerous blood fats.

women and heart disease

The general feeling is that women's risk of CVD has increased in recent years because of their increasingly hectic and unhealthy lifestyles. While it is thought that the hormone oestrogen offers women protection against heart disease until after the menopause, increased levels of stress, smoking and alcohol intake are cancelling out this protective factor. Recently it has also been found that HRT doesn't offer significant protection against heart disease during or after the menopause.

cancer

Each year around 260,000 people in the UK get cancer and 150,000 die, but expert opinion is that up to 70% of all cancers could be prevented with lifestyle changes. Smoking accounts for about 30%, while diet is thought to cause 35%.

The World Health Organization's World Cancer Report (2003) said that cancer-inducing lifestyle factors include alco-

heart facts ● Aspirin offers double protection against heart disease, by helping prevent blood clots from forming and by stopping inflammation in the arteries. ● Women with diabetes are five times as likely to have heart disease as non-diabetics – the relative risk for diabetic men is lower.

hol intake, lack of exercise, obesity and low intake of fruit and vegetables. Other probable causes include infectious diseases, a negative outlook (which may compromise the immune system) and exposure to heavy metals in the atmosphere and food.

In mid life, three of the most common cancers are of the breast, prostate (see opposite) and lung. Lung cancer is mainly caused by tobacco smoking or passive smoking and it is never too late to give up – your risk of getting cancer begins to reduce almost immediately you stop, and continues to reduce until after fifteen years your risk is no greater than that of someone who has never smoked. A diet rich in fruit and vegetables may help to protect against lung cancer and a US study found that selenium supplementation caused a 50% drop in deaths from lung cancer. Selenium is found in high quantities in Brazil nuts. See also Section 1.

Breast cancer, affecting one in ten UK women at some point in their lives (mostly 50-plus), is 25% genetic, 75% influenced by lifestyle. The two main risk factors are obesity (which increases the body's circulating oestrogens) and high alcohol intake, while HRT doubles the risk. There may be a link with the trend to have fewer babies, as women's exposure to high oestrogen levels are reduced with pregnancy and breast feeding.

A healthy diet, low in saturated fat and with a high content of plant foods, including soya, no more than 1–2 alcoholic drinks daily, adequate exercise and relaxation may all help prevent breast cancer. All women over 50 – and all with a history of breast cancer in the family – should get an annual check-up.

diabetes

Type-2 diabetes, and its frequent precursor, insulin resistance (caused by a diet high in simple carbohydrates, sugar and calories), are the modern 'plagues'. Diabetes affects nearly 1.5 million people in the UK, most in middle age and above. In the long term, it can cause heart disease, blindness and death. Lifestyle is again a very important factor in minimizing the risk of diabetes, weight control being the most obvious. A BMI above 26 in middle-aged men trebles the risk, while one over 30 increases risk by a factor of nine (more if surplus weight is carried, mostly around the waist). Again the prescription is regular exercise, watching calories, fat and sugar intake, and eating plenty of fruit, veg, fish and pulses.

prostate cancer

Prostate is the number-one cancer in males, affecting 1 in 12 men, with 12% of total UK cancer deaths per annum – although 50% of diagnosed men survive longer than 15 years. Diet is an important factor in prevention or containing the disease.

- Lycopene, the antioxidant phytochemical found in highest quantities in tomatoes (absorbed best when the tomatoes are cooked) can cut the risk by a third, and onions and onion family members, such as leeks and garlic, may also be protective.

- Broccoli, Brussels sprouts and other leafy greens contain phytochemicals called indoles which suppress prostate cancer growth by inhibiting hormones that can provoke it.

- Supplements of the mineral selenium over time also reduce the risk of developing the disease.

- It may also be wise to keep animal fat intake low, eat only moderate amounts of dairy produce, and avoid smoked, cured and charred foods.

- Other lifestyle factors that can minimize the risk include frequent sexual intercourse (which helps to clear cancer-causing chemicals via the semen), moderate intake of red wine (it is thought the phenols it contains inhibit the growth of prostate cancer cells).

- Many men are now being offered female HRT patches to reduce testosterone production – which can encourage the growth of the cancer cells.

alcohol and drugs Alcohol ... cigarettes ... cannabis ... over 90% of us rely on – or use frequently – at least one addictive substance to help us through life.

alcohol

Spending on alcohol in the UK is £30 billion a year, and research company Datamonitor believes that 60% of adults drink to cope with stress, to help them unwind and to cope with problems.

In mid life, alcohol tends to be a fixed factor in most people's lives, having been there for perhaps 30 or 40 years. Although research shows that few people admit that their alcohol intake gives them cause for concern, in fact many would prefer to be less beholden to the 'cup that cheers'.

It is true that there are a few benefits to be gained from moderate alcohol intake. The list – often cited as reason enough to carry on drinking – includes protection from heart attack, dementia, stroke and viral infections (particularly with moderate intake of red wine). It is thought that the plant chemicals such as polyphenols that alcoholic drinks often contain may have an antioxidant effect.

According to research, however, drinking in moderation is three times as beneficial for men as for women, and the protective effects of alcohol are more likely to benefit men over the age of 55 and women over 65. For these effects to be apparent, men need drink only 8 units of alcohol a week and women only three.

The negative aspects of alcohol consumption over the recommended limit of 21–28 units a week for men and 14–21 for women include increased risk of high blood pressure and cardiovascular disease for heavy drinkers, of liver disease which may lead to cirrhosis, of some cancers (in women, there is a 6% increase in risk of breast cancer for every extra alcohol unit consumed a day), of ulcers, gastritis and pancreatitis, of gout and memory loss.... and, of course, weight gain. Half a bottle of wine a day contains about 300 calories, which could put 32lb of fat on you in the course of a year if in addition to your normal energy requirements.

High alcohol intake may also effect eyesight and cause gum infections, dehydration, palpitations, muscular pains, accidents around the home and while driving, and is linked with insomnia, increased divorce, unreliability at work and depression. Plus you get hangovers. Makes you think, doesn't it? Use the tips here to cut down to a safe level. See pages 236–7 for contacts.

tobacco and drugs

The potential dangers of tobacco are well documented – it is the cause of the majority of cases of lung cancer and is one of the major contributors to heart disease and stroke. Despite this, if you have smoked for many years, giving up in mid life isn't easy.

The best course of action is to see your doctor, who may recommend a variety of nicotine replacement therapy (NRT) or Zyban – trials show that smokers are twice as likely to succeed in giving up if they use these methods. Willpower alone is often not enough, but it can be done. Use some of the tactics described for reducing alcohol intake.

If you do manage to give up, within 20 minutes of your last cigarette, blood pressure drops, within 8 hours your oxygen blood levels improve, within 2 days your taste buds begin to return, then lung capacity improves. In 5 years, your risk of dying is half of what it would have been if you had continued smoking. Smokers can reduce the risks and improve the health of the lungs by eating a healthy diet high in fish and fish oils and in fruit and vegetables, which are rich in antioxidants, especially vitamin C.

Ex-smokers tend to put on about half a stone after quitting – this is partly because of the rebirth of the taste buds, partly because snacking is used to replace the act of lighting a cigarette, and partly because nicotine raises the metabolic rate. Being a few pounds heavier is acceptable, healthwise, as a swap for giving up, but you can limit weight gain by eating sensibly and taking plenty of exercise (see Sections 1 and 2).

Cannabis and other so-called 'recreational drugs' are a common part of the social scene for young adults – and there are plenty of people in their 50s and 60s who have been using drugs since the '60s and '70s. In the long term, doctors now believe that cannabis smoking is as dangerous as nicotine, and is also linked with an increased risk of mental illness and memory problems. The relaxing effects contribute after prolonged use to a 'laid-back' mentality, where ideas are not carried through and motivation is lacking. In other words, if you want to make the most of your new mid life, cannabis is not really a friend. Take note of the tips already given for cutting back on alcohol and cigarettes.

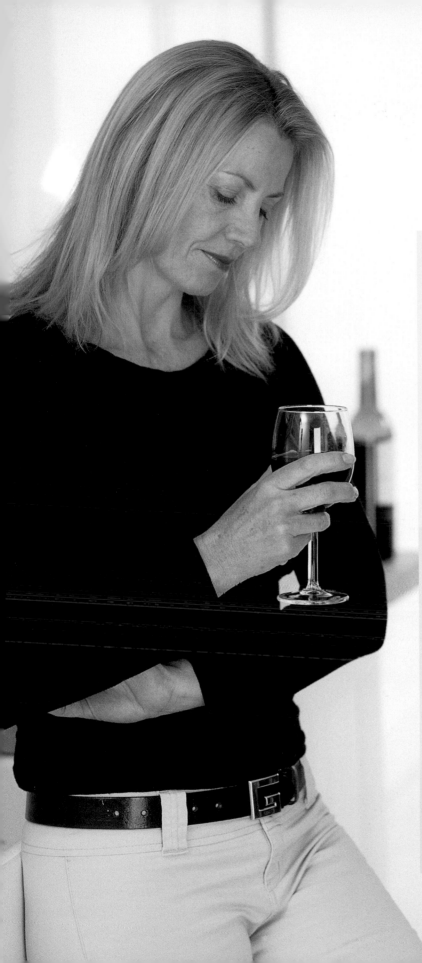

cutting down on alcohol

- Write a list of all the reasons you want to cut down/give up.

- Work out how much you are spending on alcohol a week/year and decide on something you would really like to do with that money instead. For instance, £30 a week translates to a really good holiday or a weekly massage.

- Work out how much time you spend choosing alcohol and drinking it, and think of what you could do with that time instead. An hour a day equates to a day's work a week saved, or the time you can never find to write that novel.

- Drink slowly – put your glass down between sips. Have plenty of water to quench thirst before you start drinking. Alternate an alcoholic drink with a non-alcoholic one. If you like white wine, a spritzer (half soda water, tonic or sparkling mineral water) will help.

- Buy wine and beer with lower alcohol content. Wines, especially, are much stronger than they used to be – a percentage alcohol content of 13–14% is now almost typical. This would give a total of 10.5 units for a bottle of 14% wine or over 2 units for a 150ml glass.

- If you use alcohol to relax, try other means – walking, yoga, meditation or music.

- When trying to cut down, avoid situations that make you want a drink.

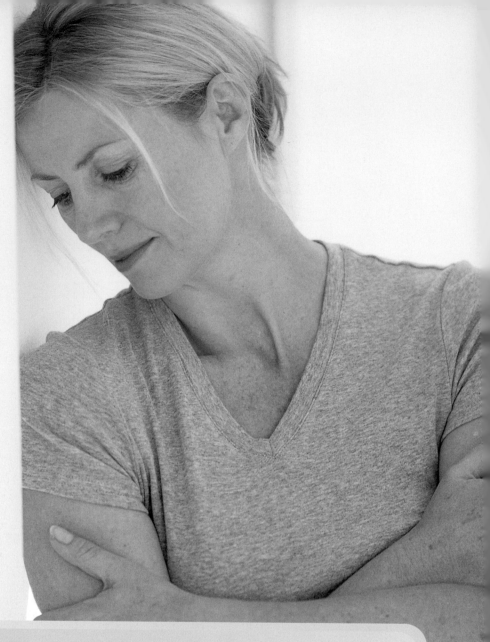

mind matters

Most of us suffer from periods of stress, depression, anxiety or brain overload from time to time, but if they are too frequent or long-lasting, this can truly affect the quality of your life. This chapter explores the solutions that could work for you.

For many people, mid life is a time when a lot of the negative feelings of youth — shyness, lack of confidence, excessive worrying over trifles, for example — have faded and been replaced with more positivity, increased self-worth and the comforting feeling that we 'know who we are' and know our place in the world.

However, it is still easy for life to run out of control when we least expect it, causing us to have to rethink what makes us happy, what makes us sad — what makes our mind work well or what causes it to show signs of breaking down. For other people, it is that very feeling of being 'in a rut', dependable, responsible, or may be even 'left behind' that makes us feel miserable. 'Going nowhere syndrome' is understandably the cause of much depression.

Stress also isn't the preserve of the young. For some in their 40s and 50s, even if we may be not achieving a lot in terms of personal progress but are still nurturing others, it can take up a lot of time, effort and energy to do so, and leave us hanging on like leaves in a storm. Anxiety over the 'typical' problems of mid life, such as divorce, redundancy or bereavement, can also be hard to cope with. Sometimes there may be no obvious cause for mental or emotional problems. Then, altering simple lifestyle factors can often change your mood or affect your mental health.

These pages will help you decide whether your mind problems are worthy of concern. Short questionnaires are provided — test yourself to find out if you are suffering from too many of the signs of depression, anxiety or stress. If so, use the tips on improving your outlook and situation. Finally, we help you to tune up your memory and conserve your brain power, summarizing all the latest advice on retaining mental agility for years to come.

depression is one of the most common complaints of all, suffered by nearly everyone at some point in their lives. One of the most difficult thing is recognizing it and admitting to it.

Depression affects 24% of women around the menopause, and a quarter of men between the ages of 55 and 65. Being depressed not only feels horrible but can adversely affect your health – research shows that depressed people's immune system is lowered, causing them to get more coughs and colds. Profound periods of depression may even help to cause early death through cancer and cardiovascular disease, researchers at the Danish Epidemiology Science Centre have found.

Though a tendency to depression can be hereditary, it is often 'circumstantial', following a bereavement, disappointment or other negative life event. It can also be hormonal (e.g. in women, before a period or during the menopause). Other causes of depression have been named as using the computer for more than five hours a day, lack of exercise, boredom, lack of sunlight (seasonal affective disorder/SAD) and some illnesses – thyroid disease can cause a depressive-like state, for instance.

In chronic depression, the balance of brain chemicals is altered and treatment via prescription drugs (usually SSRIs, see page 176) may be necessary to restore the status quo, but there are several self-help methods to help you overcome it. Getting started is the hardest step, as depression can leave you unwilling to even get out of bed.

Research shows that depressed people do best at first with gentle exercise in a non-competitive environment – swimming or yoga are ideal. Three 30-minute sessions a week of walking lead to a greater boost in mood than SSRIs, one study found.

Comfort eating is a cliché – but some foods and supplements can help to boost feelings of well-being. A generally healthy diet, high in complex carbohydrates (see Section 1), ensures good brain function, while any serotonin-boosting food (see page 189) will help. Depression can be linked with folate and selenium deficiency – eat plenty of folate-rich foods, such as leafy greens and fortified breakfast cereals, and find selenium in Brazil nuts and offal. Avoid drowning your sorrows in alcohol as this can actually lower your mood further.

Supplements of St John's Wort are mild anti-depressants, while 5-HTP and omega-3 fish oils may also work. SAD may be alleviated by means of light therapy (using special lamps or light bulbs) – home-use equipment can be pur-chased via the Internet/mail order. Essential oils and perfumes can lift mood – citrus, neroli, green tea and rosemary are uplifting. Upbeat music is a great mood-enhancer, especially if you dance – not just listen – and laughter produces body chemicals that enhance mood. Of course, you don't feel like laughing when you are depressed – but ask someone to bring you in a comedy video or book and you might find yourself laughing nonetheless.

If depression lasts longer than two weeks – see your doctor.

signs of depression

The more ticks, the more likely it is that you are depressed.

- Loss of interest in the activities that you normally enjoy.
- Low energy levels.
- Poor concentration.
- Low self-esteem.
- Crying easily.
- Inability to make decisions.
- Excessive need for sleep OR insomnia.
- Feelings of hopelessness.
- Low libido.
- Suicidal/self-harm thoughts.

anxiety is described by the British Medical Association as 'intense apprehension that may or may not have an obvious cause' and the most common form – persistent anxiety state – is most likely to begin in mid life, affecting more women than men.

Temporary anxiety is a normal and useful reaction to situations that may be harmful to us, so that we are better prepared to deal with them. For example, you feel nervous because you see a bull approaching your footpath, so you move away; you feel anxious because your report is due to be filed in an hour, so you work harder. There is also good research that shows bursts of anxiety can actually boost the immune system. However, frequent bouts for no real reason, or a permanent state of nervousness, can wreck lives.

Some people seem to have a naturally more nervous disposition than others, which is probably genetic. Such people are likely to be slim and energetic, rarely still. That heightened state of anxiety compared with the laid-back, slower neighbour only matters if it matters to you. Persistent anxiety state (PAS) is the term for when you have excessive, frequent/long-term anxiety that you can't control, while panic disorder consists of bouts of intense anxiety combined with physical symptoms, which may occur even when there is little to worry about.

Sometimes PAS may include panic disorder. With panic disorder, it is advisable to see your doctor, who may refer you for cognitive behaviour therapy (CBT) and/or medication. Persistent anxiety may also need medical help, and can also benefit from CBT but there are several ways you may be able to help yourself.

Relaxation exercises, such as deep breathing, meditation, stretching, yoga (see Section 2), can calm anxiety. For short-term nerves (e.g. before a stage performance), high-energy exercise is best – for example, skipping. Massage can relax the mind and reduce anxiety. Calming music or sounds (e.g. chill-out or waves) work for short-term anxiety. Focusing on situations that worry you and picturing yourself dealing with them in a positive successful way are useful.

Hypnotherapy with a trained consultant helps some people and is especially helpful if your anxiety is specific and short-term (e.g. giving a speech) or is phobia-based (e.g. fear of spiders). The supplement relora (extract of magnolia) has been shown in clinical trials to reduce anxiety and stress. Remember that short-term worry in itself is fairly harmless – what may do the damage is anxiety about worrying.

signs of anxiety

The more you can tick, the more likely it is that you have a high level of anxiety.

- Sense of foreboding with no obvious reason.
- Inability to relax physically.
- Brain won't slow down or unwind, particularly at bedtime.
- Insomnia.
- Inability to concentrate on a book, film, newspaper article.
- Worrying thoughts which won't go away.
- Abdominal cramps, nausea.
- Loose bowels.
- Frequent visits to the loo to urinate.
- Perspiration, hot flushes.
- Trembling hands.
- Difficulty in swallowing.
- Shortness of breath or dizziness.
- Palpitations.

The top 10 things we worry about Money, personal health, work performance, losing our job/retirement, health of family, relationships, getting older, the way we look, not being fit/slim; the world around us.

stress might be defined as unacceptable pressures inflicted on you in the short or long term which result in a wide range of potentially negative physical and emotional reactions.

All of us feel stress at some time, which is normal and can actually be productive and good for us. When we are stressed, hormones such as adrenaline, are released to increase arousal, energy, strength and performance, thus helping us get through busy periods or difficult things.

In modern life, though, stress can easily become overwhelming and/or the normal state, and it is then that we may need to find ways to reduce it. Long-term living under constant stress, whether physical or mental, can exacerbate, or is linked with, all the following conditions: high blood pressure (due to increased heartbeat), central fat distribution (big belly, due to extra circulating cortisol, the 'stress hormone'), both of which increase the risk of cardiovascular disease; digestive disorders, such as ulcers, constipation and irritable bowel syndrome; insomnia; reliance on alcohol or drugs; impotence; muscular pain; burn-out/nervous breakdown, impaired memory and a variety of mental disorders. Stress can also affect the immune system and leave you more prone to infection and even cancer.

These effects can be more frequent or more apparent for people in mid life who have been under stress for many years, so if you feel that you are stressed out then it is time to take action to reduce the stress and/or help your body to cope.

coping with stress

A healthy diet will provide all the vitamins and minerals your body needs to help it cope with stress. Particularly important are vitamin C and B group, which are depleted more quickly under stress and can't be stored in the body.

Supplements of zinc, magnesium and echinacea will help boost the immune system against stress-induced illness; a diet high in antioxidants will help repair the free-radical damage caused by long-term stress, and you could also try relora (extract of magnolia) to help you through short-term

high-stress periods. For stress that is based on anger, frustration or any emotion, exercise is vital – short bursts of intense interval training (or even plate-smashing), with plenty of rest in between, are good, but any kind of physical activity will help to disperse adrenaline and cortisol.

Physical contact, such as stroking, massage or touching, has been shown to produce hormones called oxytocins which reduce stress, especially in women. Short-term stress-relievers include good sex, 'palming' your eyes with your hands, yawning, stretching, or a cup of camomile tea.

Get enough sleep (see pages 188–9). Never work more than 4 hours at one sitting/9 hours in

signs of stress

The more you tick, the more likely you are suffering from stress.

- You work more than forty-five hours a week.
- You easily 'fly off the handle' or exhibit grumpiness.
- You are sometimes irrational.
- You have a poor memory.
- You have trouble concentrating.
- You jump out of your skin at a sudden noise.
- You have insomnia.
- You have a lot of fat around your abdomen.
- You feel exhausted much of the time, and no better in the mornings.
- You frequently have an upset stomach.
- You regularly use alcohol and/or drugs.
- You often feel that you are about to 'crack up'.
- You have low libido.
- You sometimes get chest pains but you have no heart condition.
- Your muscles often ache or hurt and/or you often feel stiff.
- You get dizzy spells.
- You often cancel social engagements or have little time for friends.
- You succumb to a lot of small illnesses and often feel unwell.

Mr Grumpy? It's all in the hormones ● Irritability is a sign of stress – and research (admittedly on sheep!) shows that declining testosterone levels increase irritability. See Andropause (pages 174, 177) ● Scientists have found a gene, 5-HTT, which has two versions, one sensitive, the other coping. Depending on which our DNA has, we may cope well with stress or succumb to it. So don't feel guilty, blame your genes instead!

one day. Learn to say no to people and stop trying to be an all-people pleaser. Plan for 15 minutes' total peace and quiet once every day, or in three 5-minute sessions (excluding sleep time). Maintain a balance between home, work, family and friends.

Alzheimer's disease

People with poor memory in mid life or younger don't necessarily go on to get Alzheimer's disease, but forgetfulness is the first-stage sign. Alzheimer's is a degenerative brain disease that causes nerve cells to die off, so the brain shrinks and its structure and chemical content changes character. It affects half a million people in the UK, most over 65, but research has shown that people in their 50s with high blood pressure and high cholesterol levels are 2.5 times as likely to develop the disease.

Very modest drinking of alcohol (up to 1 unit a day) may help prevent dementia, while regular drinking of more than 1 unit actually increases the risk. Poor blood supply to the brain (often caused by atherosclerosis/hardening of the arteries) is thought to increase the risk too – regular aerobic exercise, avoidance of smoking, a diet low in saturated fat and high in fish oils, fruit and vegetables can counteract this, and gingko biloba may also help by keeping the arteries connected to the brain supple and free from clogging. Folic acid supplements lower the blood concentration of homocysteine – high levels of this amino acid double the risk of Alzheimer's, it has been found.

Aspirin or other anti-inflammatory drugs (NSAIDs), taken daily over a long period, lower the risk by 70%. HRT for post-menopausal women and THT (testosterone treatment) for men may also lower the risk, although this is yet to be proved. There is also still debate over whether aluminium (in drinking water and/or from aluminium pans) may be linked, as Alzheimer's seems to be most common in areas with highest levels of aluminium in the water.

memory

In mid life, many people complain that their memory is much worse than it was even a few years ago. Powers of memory, mental flexibility and reasoning are associated with the frontal lobes of the brain, the power of which tends to decline as we age. This decline can be kept at bay with a variety of strategies. (Further advice on maintaining brain power appears in the next section).

● Some supplements can help. In tests, Siberian ginseng improved information storage and retrieval; gingko biloba may aid memory by improving blood flow to the brain; soya isoflavones may boost receptors in the hippocampus (the brain's memory area); phosphatidyl serine improves the action of brain neurotransmitters and may slow memory decline.

● Poor memory is a symptom of thyroid disorder – get yourself checked out if you also have tiredness, constipation and/or feel cold all the time.

● Oily fish or fish oil supplements may help boost memory.

● Memory loss can be associated with depression, stress and anxiety.

● People with a high IQ and/or who have intellectual stimulation and an active social life generally suffer less from memory loss.

● Folic acid supplements lower blood levels of the amino acid homocysteine – high levels double the risk of Alzheimer's. As with poor memory, keeping the brain active will help stave off Alzheimer's.

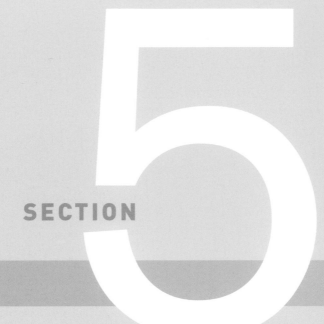

SECTION

5

time for your
newlife

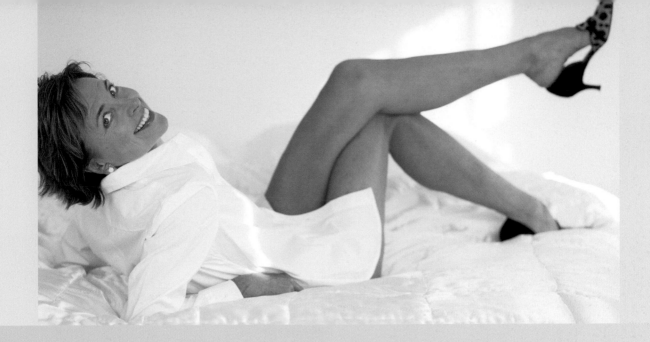

Who are you now? The earlier years of mid life are so tremendously busy for most of us that you may – when there is eventually a breathing space – suddenly realize that you have no idea who you really are any more, it has been so long since you had the time or energy to think about your own needs.

As our allotted life span gets longer and longer, most of us are hardly more than halfway through our lives when we get to 50 or so. How will you spend the thirty, forty or fifty years you may have ahead? Do you know what you want to do?

Mid life is an ideal time for making changes and choices, for finding new roles to play, for getting in touch with the present and making plans for the future. And yet, often none of that happens. All too frequently we settle for cosy familiarity or, worse, resign ourselves to what life is, rather than what it could be.

But we all must change and move on, whether we like it or not. And change is what helps to keep us young and enthusiastic. Section 5 helps you to get the most out of your life, and to answer that question – Who are you now?

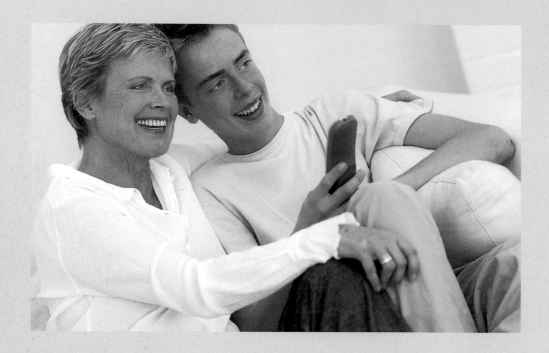

so you have good health, a good diet, good looks and a fit body What are you going to do with it all?

While a typical young person tends to grab opportunities as they speed by – and feels that a year in a job is an aeon; that 'new' is good and 'old' is less good – one of the most common markers of passing youth has often been seen as a growing reluctance to change in ideas, direction, lifestyle or character; to hang on to what is there; to accept that this is 'the beginning of the end'.

In recent decades, however, we have realized that mid life is the end of nothing, but a new start. It is time to 'go for it' – whatever 'it' may be. Indeed, research shows that it is people who embrace innovation gladly and who lead what is always termed a 'full and active life' who live longer, and appear younger than their years.

Of course, there are parts of your life that you are right not to want to change and would, indeed, be foolish so to do – a happy marriage, for instance. And there is nothing wrong with being quiet and contemplative, enjoying your own company or not wanting to move from the home you've lived in for the past twenty years. These are your strong and stable foundations – recognizing them as such but not being frightened to add new elements are what will always make you feel alive.

Section 5 helps you to decide what it is that you really want, and to deal with times in your life when matters are decided for you.

The first chapter of the section, Making It Your Way, is, if you like, the sly kick to make you take that slightly frightening leap of faith, or sometimes the gently encouraging friend – which is often all you need. It is full of ideas and decision-making tools.

Of course, there are a lot of things you can't change – a death in the family, for example, or a job redundancy. The Letting Go chapter offers advice on dealing with change that is forced upon you, and looks at the difficult period when the children 'fly the nest'.

Streamline Your Life is where we appraise your time, and how you use it. Mid life can often be more 'time-poor' than any other period, so there is help with organizing your days and forward-planning. We also consider how to keep your brain sharp and efficient. Many people have to make a decision about whether to work or retire, whether to commute or work from home – we help you weigh up the options.

Finally we look at your changing relationship with your family and friends, your elderly relatives and your social life. Some people say that the only real friends you ever make are when you are young ... but, as we shall see, that is simply not true.

It really is time for your new life now – let's get going.

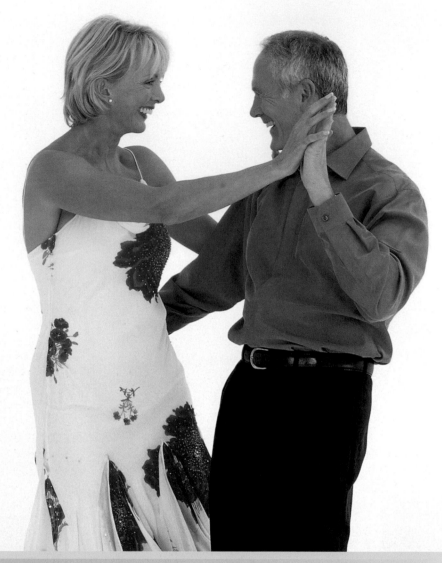

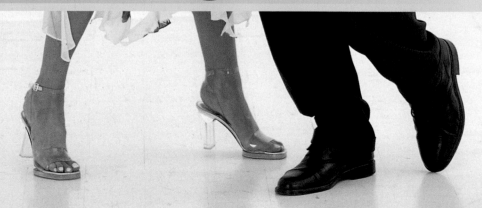

making it your way

If you can't do what you want now, today, this week, this year – when can you do it? Mid life is not only the best but also the most important time to find yourself, be yourself, please yourself and enjoy yourself. And that doesn't actually mean you have to change into an extremely selfish person, or feel guilty.

Life at any age is all about balance, but too often during the busy, busy years of the 20s, 30s and often 40s your own needs, pleasures and concerns have to take a back seat. You tend to put yourself last. Women, in particular those mixing career with family, are adept at doing this, but it is by no means a female preserve. Many men work long hours for perhaps a large salary but little other reward and still have to play many roles at home – protector, DIY expert, gardener, chef, whatever – as well.

So, when you reach the late 40s or 50s you need and deserve to recognize that your own life is as important as anyone else's. The people you know and love should actually benefit from your recognition of this fact (though they may take a while to realize it!).

Given the modern gift of a period of many years after the age of 50 of reasonable health and comparative wealth and free time, it really IS time to be your own person. So in this chapter we look at all the ways you might make some changes and choices that will, hopefully, have you feeling more content, more alive and happier than you have been for some time. In mid life many people make changes only when forced to by a 'wake-up call', but often when this happens we find that we wish we had made those changes a long time ago.

First, do the questionnaire overleaf to find out how much of a rut you are in, then use the idea on the following pages to help you decide how things might improve. From enjoying your new place in the 'pecking order', to seeking anything from tranquillity to excitement, there is plenty of choice.

All it takes is some self-belief and confidence to dig out what you really want and work out how to get it. Go on – why NOT cram in a few detours, adventures and challenges, rather than later having to ponder on what might have been?

are you in a rut?

Answer the following 10 questions honestly, choosing the answer that most nearly matches your experience if there isn't one that is exactly right, then calculate whether you have ticked more As, more Bs or more Cs, and check your profile below.

1 how long is it since you cooked a new recipe?
a) 1 week or less.
b) 1–3 months.
c) Around a year.

2 how often do you buy yourself something new to wear?
a) Every month or less.
b) Twice a year.
c) Hardly ever.

3 how often do you look at a daily newspaper different from your regular one?
a) Once a week or less.
b) Now and then.
c) Never.

4 when did you last have a weekend away from home not related to work?
a) Within the last 2 months.
b) Within the last 6 months.
c) Rarely have weekends away.

5 when choosing your major annual holiday, which of these options do you go for?
a) Go to a new country every year.
b) Go to the same area but in different accommodation.
c) Always go to the same resort and same accommodation.

6 tv – do you have the following?
a) Satellite TV with all the stations.
b) Satellite but only the basic free channels.
c) BBC, ITV, Channel 4, Five.

7 how long is it since you made friends with anyone new?
a) This last year.
b) 2–3 years.
c) More than 5 years.

8 when did you last voluntarily do something that made you feel a bit nervous, afraid or unsure?
a) Within the last 2 months.
b) Within the last year.
c) Can't remember.

9 how long is it since you learned a new skill (e.g. hobby/language) not related to work?
a) Within the last year.
b) Within the last 5 years.
c) Can't remember.

10 what is your view of the Internet?
a) Great – use it all the time.
b) We have a computer but I don't really know what I am doing.
c) Don't like the idea, don't have a computer.

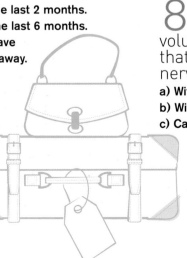

scoring

Mostly As: You are most certainly not in a rut – don't lose your sense of adventure as you get older, it is what keeps people feeling young and living longer. The UK Wellbeing Survey 2002 found that it is boredom, more than stress or lack of money, that diminishes a sense of well-being as we age.

Mostly Bs: That rut is looking dangerously close and you have one foot in it. You're in danger of stagnating, so it is time to reinvent areas of your life and see what adventures are out there for the taking.

Mostly Cs: Oh dear! You fell into a rut a while ago and you can't seem to get yourself out – perhaps you don't even think you want to. But you need to get up and dust yourself off. As they say – this is no rehearsal, this is your life.

So – did my little questionnaire show that you ARE in a rut, or borderline? It is surprising how infrequently many of us even bother to think about what we do each day as we get older. We just get up and get on with today much as we did yesterday. If nothing awful happens, then it is a good day.

There is, however, more to your life than that. Sometimes you need to be brave and bold to change things, that's all. You have that capacity. Indeed, new research in the UK by the British Household Panel shows that, while in the past people over the age of 41 rarely made voluntary major changes to their lives, now we are actually more willing to change jobs, households, partners or lifestyles than ever before.

You may feel you don't have the time … that life is far too busy to worry about making changes that could cost effort and stress you out even more. So if time is your problem, go to pages 222–7 for help. If you do have time, however, start thinking and planning now about how you would like your life to be. You need to make this time and make sure you are focused on your thoughts. Take a walk on your own to begin, or sit in a quiet room in a comfortable chair. If you are going to write ideas down, use a pen and some paper, not the computer. Build yourself some mental pictures as you take these 3 steps.

redefine your base
See what you already have and take a fresh new look at it. Family. Work. Home. How are you coping with changes in the pecking order? Once your children grow up you have a different role to play (see Family and Friendships, pages 228–35). Accept that things do change and you need to change with them (for more on this, see Letting Go, pages 216–21).

Make a list of all the things in your life that make you happy, that you don't want to change. This defines what you have achieved in life so far and gives you a good springboard. Try to recall when you were a child – the wonder and joy you felt at quite ordinary things, sometimes just at the simple fact of being alive. And think about the importance of keeping an open mind to opinions and possibilities.

find the right balance
This is such a terrific time to get balance back into your life after what has probably been a mad few years. Apart from health, balance is probably the most important factor in living a happy and long life. Think back to when you were a young adult. What were your hopes, dreams and ambitions then? How many got forgotten or pushed aside? We all have wishes that we never fulfilled; some will no longer be what we want at all, while some can be still be achieved.

Ask yourself some questions about how much of the following you have in your life:
● Peace ● Excitement? ● Innovation?
● Friends? ● A close family? ● Culture?
● Information? ● Beauty? ● Challenge?
● Spirituality? ● Work? ● Leisure?

See if you can pinpoint areas where you could get more; areas that are too much. Think about how you can create or restore balance.

make plans
Now it is time to make lists and plans. The discussion overleaf on retirement may help you decide on the right work/leisure balance for you. The ideas on pages 214–15 may give you some inspiration for different things to do with your time.

Write your own list of things you want to do. Divide the list into three – Big Things (e.g. start your own business from home; write that best-selling novel), Little or Medium Things (e.g. call up some old friends, decorate the kitchen), and Self-improvement Things (e.g. learn a new language, try to stop being so negative). Discuss the list with your partner, if you have one.

Finally, make a plan of how, when and where you are going to do these things. I would suggest making this plan realistic. If you have brought up a family or run any kind of business, you will know how to make schedules that can be kept to.

Pick a few 'big', 'little' and 'self-improvement' things to do in the next year. Look at the plan – is there a good mix? Pin it up somewhere. Start on one thing from each of the three sections straight away. Don't rely on things happening without you making them happen. Research shows that people create their own luck . Those who think of themselves as 'lucky' tend to be optimists who exploit opportunities and listen to their own intuition.

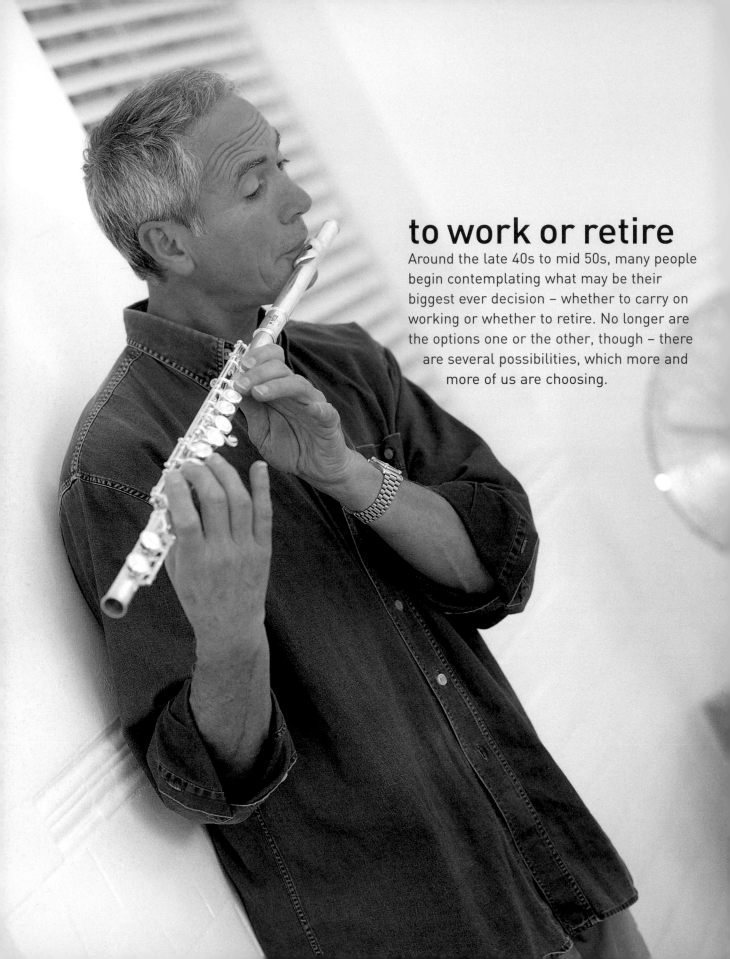

to work or retire

Around the late 40s to mid 50s, many people begin contemplating what may be their biggest ever decision – whether to carry on working or whether to retire. No longer are the options one or the other, though – there are several possibilities, which more and more of us are choosing.

full retirement

This is no longer always unavoidable at 60 or 65, as it was for so long for so many of us. In most careers, whether high-flying or undemanding, you no longer have to be 'pensioned off' (what a horrible term!) at a certain age if you don't want to be. Many people choose to carry on working, not just because of the extra money but because they enjoy work and/or are worried that there won't be much in life for them if they do retire.

However, when – inevitably – retirement is impending, for many people it really does seem to spell 'the end', with little left to look forward to except physical decline. If you dread the thought of retiring, first banish the 'R' word from your vocabulary. Instead think of yourself as being allowed to start afresh. Try not to be afraid, try not to avoid thinking about the moment, and do what those who are happy to retire do – plan ahead. Open your mind to possibilities, start making lists as early as possible beforehand and don't discount anything or anyone who may enrich your 'retirement' years. See the panel on the right for ideas on other work you can do.

If you don't want to – or are not able to – carry on working and yet still don't feel happy to retire, it may be because you feel your home life or partner relationship is poor or unfulfilling. In that case, read Family and Friendships, pages 228–35.

redundancy

This can be worse mentally than normal-age retirement, even if cushioned with a payoff. Check out the panel on the right for ideas on how to get back into work mode.

choosing to retire

One UK survey of working women found that their main causes of stress were work-related: 51% cited heavy workload, 42% lack of leisure time, 34% trouble-making work colleagues and 21% bad bosses/employees. No wonder that many women can't

new ways of working

If you don't want to carry on in your old job in the same way, but you don't really want to go for full retirement, weigh up some of these options:

- **go part-time** or job share.
- **see if you can do your job from home** either full time or at least on certain days of the week.
- **take a gap year** then return to your old job – more and more 40+ people are doing this. One way to fund it is to rent out your home for the year.
- **try seasonal** or voluntary work.
- **apply for a new job** Many people do find new employment whatever their age. A survey reveals that 50% of retired people who later decide to go to work again get a job with no problem.
- **retrain** The largest percentage of students returning to education in adulthood are women over 40.
- **start your own business** If you have no mortgage now, or have redundancy money or savings, or can find a sponsor, it may be time to start up a small business, whether in a similar area to your old career or on a completely new tack. Either way, it will pay you to plan ahead and not leave your old job until you have everything in place as far as possible. At least make sure you have done your research/found your gap in the market and know how you plan to make things work.
- **work from home** With communications now being so good, you can move to the country/seaside/abroad and still do a wide variety of work from home.
- **use your home** A large house might be a guest house or country hotel; a large garden might be a herb garden centre or a boarding kennels. Great cook? You could make produce to sell. Ex photographer/designer/captain of industry? You could do weekend courses in your specialist field.

the UK Wellbeing Survey 2002 found that the top five factors that effect well-being are: ● Feeling in control ● Having an optimistic outlook ● Being content with your appearance ● Having a sense of belonging in the community ● Having good relationships with family and friends. **Work didn't come into the equation at all!**

wait to retire once they are over 50! No doubt similar questioning of men – who often get work-related depression in mid life, when they may be passed over for promotion, or may be made to feel 'past it' performance-wise – would reveal similar results.

Research shows that those who have a happy retirement tend to have a family or partner rather than living on their own, and have a circle of friends (not all work comrades) and outside interests, hobbies and so on.

One of the main keys to a successful retirement seems to be – long before the actual retirement date – thinking about what you will do with your lovely new free time. Surprisingly, having a lot of money isn't one of the most important factors. A study by Imperial College, London, of 300 people between the ages of 55 and 75 found that good health and a small network of close friends were far more important than wealth in retirement. Two other studies in the UK in recent years have found similar results. It is only if annual income per head drops below £7,500 that being poor brings unhappiness, according to one of the reports.

Of course, if all your 'wish list' retirement items rely on money for fulfilment, but you are not as wealthy as you would like, then you may have a problem until you contemplate the saying, 'Money can't buy you happiness. It only helps you look for it in a lot more places.'

choosing to carry on working

Research has found that people who work past their 'official' retiring age are, not surprisingly, wealthier than people who take early or normal-age retirement. The same study also found that they tend to be healthier – three-quarters of working men aged 55–75 described their health as excellent or very good, compared with only

50% of those who had retired. However, another London-based study of 800 men found that the mental functioning of the retired men was better.

At present in the UK about 10% of the population works full time after the age of 65 (men) or 60 (women) but, although ageism is still widely practised in the workplace, more and more employers are realizing that early retirement is a waste of talent, experience, skill and expertise, and by 2006 workplace ageism will be outlawed in the UK. Perhaps the best option for people who would like to continue working over 65, but who need more leisure-related balance in their lives, is to check out other 'halfway' options – see page 213.

boredom or burn out While you may not want to give up work, you may be feeling almost terminally bored with your actual job, or you may be suffering from burnout. More and more people in their 40s and 50s are changing career, changing tack, or finding other ways out of the work rut. If you feel trapped at work for any reason, it is always best to find an exit strategy. We all need change to stir ourselves up. If you leave a job you no longer enjoy, you have lost nothing except your income. Although this can be more than scary, downsizing early can be rewarding and life-enhancing. Also see page 213 for income-generating ideas.

do something different...

10 ways to spice up your life

The Internet has details of many of the ideas mentioned here. Note that people in poor health or with a physical disability are not advised to try some of the more demanding suggestions.

1 Read your way through the Top 100 all-time favourite books (in the UK, produced by the BBC). Joining the library helps.

2 Take to the skies – depending on your fear-factor level, go hot-air-ballooning/gliding/microlighting/sky diving.

3 Do someone else a favour – whether it's a sponsored walk for charity or shopping for a sick neighbour, helping others, research shows, makes us more cheerful.

4 Book up a course of sessions with a life coach.

5 Go for a weekend camping in a tent – everyone should do it once in their lives.

6 Set yourself a physical challenge – climb Kilimanjaro, run a half-marathon, walk the Pennine Way, learn gymnastics or salsa dancing.

7 Have a spa weekend on your own, with all the treatments and a light diet.

8 Plan a home-swap vacation (you go to someone's home for your holiday and they come to yours) – it's less expensive and more fun than a hotel or apartment holiday.

9 Go to a theme park and take one of the scary rides – or at least, go on the old-fashioned carousel with the dancing horses and eat some popcorn or candy floss.

10 Go to your local train station and get on the first train that comes along (excluding local commuter trains). Go right to the end of the line and stay there for at least the day.

now think of 10 ideas of your own!

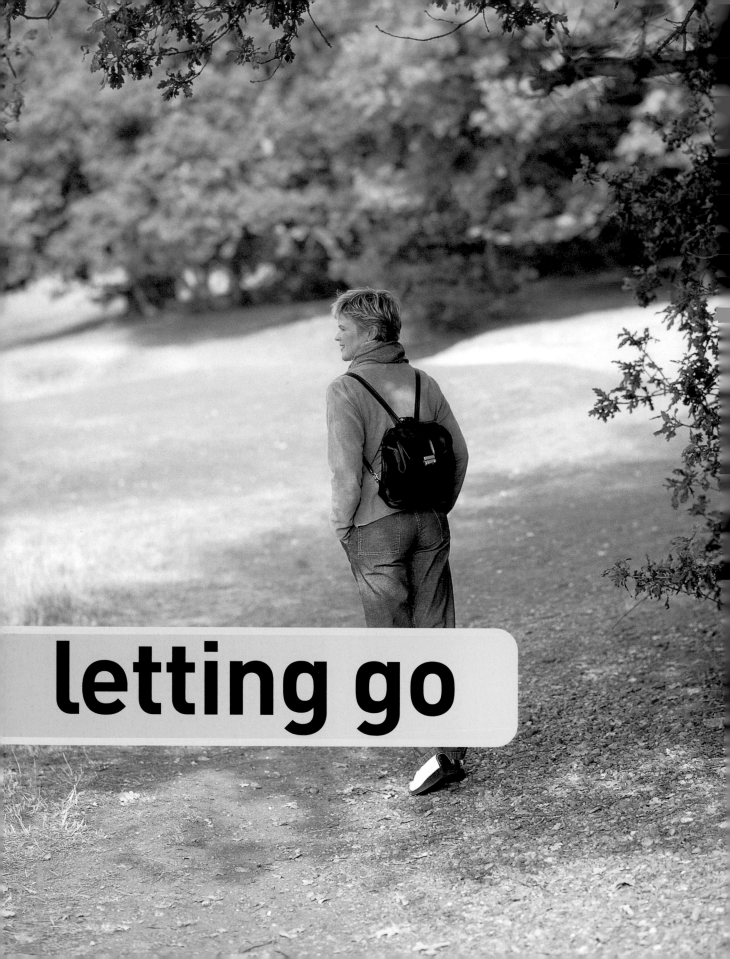

letting go

In mid life, most people face an often surprising degree of change – and not always of their own making. Learning to let go and move on is never easy, but unexpected or unwanted changes can be made less traumatic ...

Mid life is when the roots that most of us put down in early adulthood become deep and firm. Years pass by and it can be easy to get lulled into feeling that what you have – how your life is – will stay that way for ever. Often in mid life, though, a long period of equilibrium will be swiftly followed by sudden or unexpected or unwanted change. Sometimes you may see it coming, or, indeed, know it is coming, but at other times it can be a shock.

The most common of these changes are the end of a long-term marriage or relationship, children leaving home or going to university, a parent, partner or other close person dying, a job redundancy or forced early retirement, and having to move home or area.

All these changes can be – and must be – coped with, but it is rarely easy, and some of us find it harder to deal with than others. You have to learn to prepare yourself for change, and then to let go after it has happened, and move on. It may even be possible to enjoy change even though you have to face something you always thought you would dread. A change of perspective is often all you really need to wind up realizing that your life can actually improve.

This chapter discusses each of the most usual 'change' situations and how you might cope effectively.

we all have to deal with change
Some people thrive on it – even seek it out – while others fear it and attempt to avoid it. These pages offer guidance on all the major 'forced' changes you are likely to meet in mid life and suggests how you might cope with them.

a death in the family

In mid life most people face the death of a loved one – parent, partner, friend – perhaps for the first time, and with it the truth of our own mortality, the inevitability of losing people we love, and of the irreversible nature of death. Once people are gone, you can't tell them you care about them any more, and you can't say sorry. So grief is often coloured with guilt and both are hard to bear. If it is a parent who dies, you feel that sense of being orphaned just as if you were ten years old. Now it is up to you to be the 'older generation' and – as my husband said after his mother died, 'Well, it is our turn next.' And the death of a younger person – someone your own age or younger – can be an even greater shock, proving that you are not immortal.

So there is nothing positive to be gained from the experience of death. Well, perhaps there is, although it may not be apparent for some long time. People who have suffered loss often say that the death pulls them up sharp and makes them reassess their own lives. It may make you behave differently towards people you care about, may help you to live your life to the full and in the present, rather than thinking about what might have been or procrastinating.

Death can also bring you back in touch with people who were once important to you and/or make you realize how many people do care about you. Indeed, when coping with the death of a partner or other close family member, it is this support that gets most of us through. There are no short-cuts to coming to terms with the changes a death will bring to you – but letting people into your life, and not putting on a 'brave front', are the two ways to begin.

Joining a group of people who are in the same situation as you, or have recently been through it and have survived, has been shown to shorten the period of depression that follows any bereavement. The support, encouragement and advice you will receive from such a group are invaluable.

moving home

There are two main reasons why you may need to move home now. The first is that you want, or need, to downsize for reasons of finance or convenience. This often accompanies a divorce or split, or a job loss or retirement – so it can often be a double dose of misery for people who don't like change.

If finance is the reason, you need to act quickly before debts mount – and the business of selling up/finding somewhere to go/organizing everything is often a good therapy once you begin. So don't dither – grab the change and take charge. The main decision that needs careful thought is whether to stay in the same area or move away.

The worst part of moving somewhere smaller can be having to divest yourself of treasured possessions/furniture. See if you can offload these on to children, siblings or other relatives who will appreciate your things (obviously with divorce your ex will take the surplus); otherwise choose carefully what goes and what stays and recognize that a good clear-out is symbolic of what is happening in your life. You will almost certainly surprise yourself and find that this makes you feel better. If it turns out the old prints in the attic fetch a mint at auction, so much the better – time for a holiday.

You may also decide you need to move for other reasons – to get a new job, be near children/elderly parents, for instance. In such cases, the move is at least partly your decision, which does make it easier, as you have a larger element of control. So let the decision be right. You need to make a list of pros and cons of the potential move before going ahead, take all the advice you can get, and make sure everyone involved in the decision is consulted.

Once the move is done, you need to strike a balance between keeping in touch with old friends and family and making a new life. For more tips on this, see the discussion on the End of a marriage/relationship (page 220) and the chapter on Family and Friendships (pages 228–35).

career change/end

When you lose your job, for whatever reason – or perhaps are made bankrupt – there is little more confidence-damaging, as work still fundamentally defines who we are. So why is it that while some collapse in the face of what they see as disaster, perhaps becoming chronically depressed and unable to function, others cope well and emerge happier than ever before?

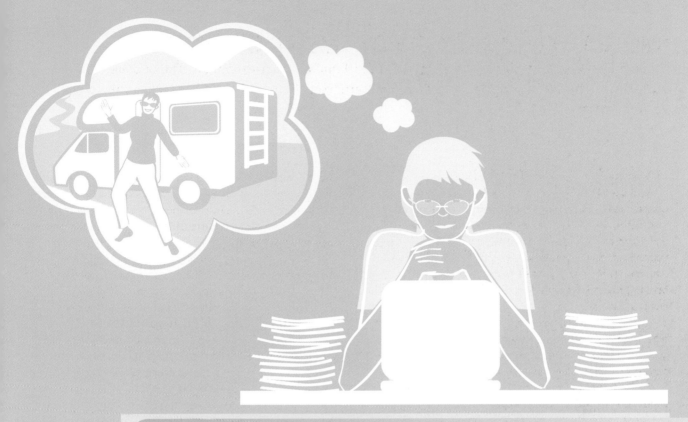

dealing with the fear of change

- Understand that life is dynamic not static, and so are people's needs. If unwanted change happens to you, it isn't necessarily anything you are doing/did wrong. Knowing that you are not at fault helps.

- Don't try to pre-empt change by not living a full life or by clinging to what you have. It won't work and it will make you feel more isolated and worse when change does happen. Take risks and make choices yourself, otherwise others will do it for you.

- Change can seem worse if you feel you have no element of control. For changes that you know will happen eventually – for example, children leaving home – get involved in the build-up to the change rather than ignoring it. For instance, helping children sort out their new lives before they leave will make you feel part of the process and not a helpless bystander.

- Visualize yourself in different situations – e.g. in a different house, without a job (if you currently have one) or living alone (if you are currently with a partner). Plan what you might do in each of these situations. Always have time each day to visualize what your life could be like. This powerful tool will help you cope if your thoughts become reality.

- For sudden change that may leave you feeling bereft or depressed, remember that you can always have professional counselling. Knowing that you have this option if anything 'bad' happens to you can be a great comfort blanket.

One important factor is having family/partner who don't/doesn't make you feel that their happiness – or your worth – is dependent upon your income. You also need your own sense of self-worth beyond that provided by your capacity to work and/or earn well. Developing this sense early in adulthood is protection against the depression of 'failure' at work. However, it is not too late to nurture it even after the event: see pages 212–14, where we discuss work and retirement. One thing is certain – it isn't too late to seek other employment, and there is little element of luck involved. Research shows that all of us can 'get lucky' if we keep optimistic and try hard enough.

end of a marriage/relationship

If your partner wants to leave you – or walks out, or even if they have an affair – research shows this is an even bigger blow to most people than losing a long-term job or business, and almost as bad as if they had died. Around 165,000 people a year get divorced in the UK, however, so it is something many of us will have to deal with – especially men, as three-quarters of proceedings are initiated by women.

There are steps you can take to ensure that your own long-term relationship doesn't end in a split (see Family and Friendships, pages 228–35). These days an affair needn't be the end of a relationship, and can even make it better (usually with the help of counselling, though). But sometimes you have to admit it just isn't going to work out, and let go. Give yourself a month for every year that you were together to come to terms with the change. Of course, this is an average – you can help yourself by making sure that you do all you can to ensure a 'good divorce'. It may be possible to split and, eventually (or even sooner), be friends.

If there are offspring, you will feel much better if you can pull off a non-acrimonious divorce. And you can help yourself avoid the loneliness that splitting often brings by keeping in touch with family and friends throughout your marriage/partnership, and by always remembering to have a life that doesn't depend on your partner for its fun or satisfaction.

The needier and more dependent you were in the partnership, the more likely it is that you will have to be taught to be

happy again – counselling, friends and family can all help you to do this and it is vital to accept help rather than pushing people away. The two most important things to learn are: if your partner is now your ex, they were a part of your life which was right for then, but not now; and although you are no longer together, what you had and shared is still important and always will be.

children leaving home

When you are a parent with children still living at home, the question, 'What shall I do today?' is rarely needed. Over a period of about twenty years, time is automatically filled with seeing to their many needs. Occasional fleeting moments of wondering what happened to the selfish life you used to lead may flicker in your brain, but that is all.

Hence, when suddenly it's all over and the last child leaves you with 'empty-nest syndrome', getting back your own life can be a tremendous shock. Then there is the awesome quiet in the house. The lack of loud music, phones ringing, teenagers laughing, shouting. Why is it that all the things you craved – the time to yourself, the peace, the return to civilization as you used to know it – no longer seem quite so appealing?

Don't worry – it may take weeks, or even months, but soon you will remember what it is you were planning to do and why you sometimes craved your own space and time. Hasten this along by not spending your days and evenings sitting by the phone waiting for offspring to ring. By not constantly phoning them yourself (learn to text them instead). By not always being available 24/7 to sort out laundry and love problems.

Fill the house with your own preferred noise, laughter and shouting by all means, but relish the peace and some selfish time. Most of us have long, long lists of things we want to do – so plan them and do them. You will always be there for your children, but the last thing they need when they leave home is to feel worried about you or, worse, guilty about you. The sooner you fill the gaps they left the better you will feel. And when they do come home or, even better, invite you round to their place, you'll all love each other all the more.

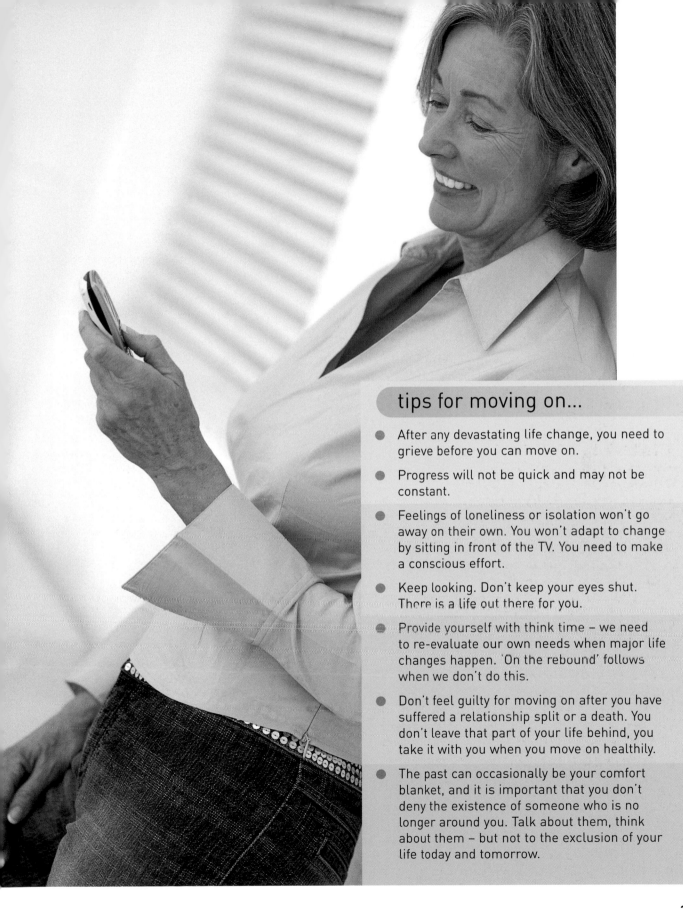

tips for moving on...

- After any devastating life change, you need to grieve before you can move on.

- Progress will not be quick and may not be constant.

- Feelings of loneliness or isolation won't go away on their own. You won't adapt to change by sitting in front of the TV. You need to make a conscious effort.

- Keep looking. Don't keep your eyes shut. There is a life out there for you.

- Provide yourself with think time – we need to re-evaluate our own needs when major life changes happen. 'On the rebound' follows when we don't do this.

- Don't feel guilty for moving on after you have suffered a relationship split or a death. You don't leave that part of your life behind, you take it with you when you move on healthily.

- The past can occasionally be your comfort blanket, and it is important that you don't deny the existence of someone who is no longer around you. Talk about them, think about them – but not to the exclusion of your life today and tomorrow.

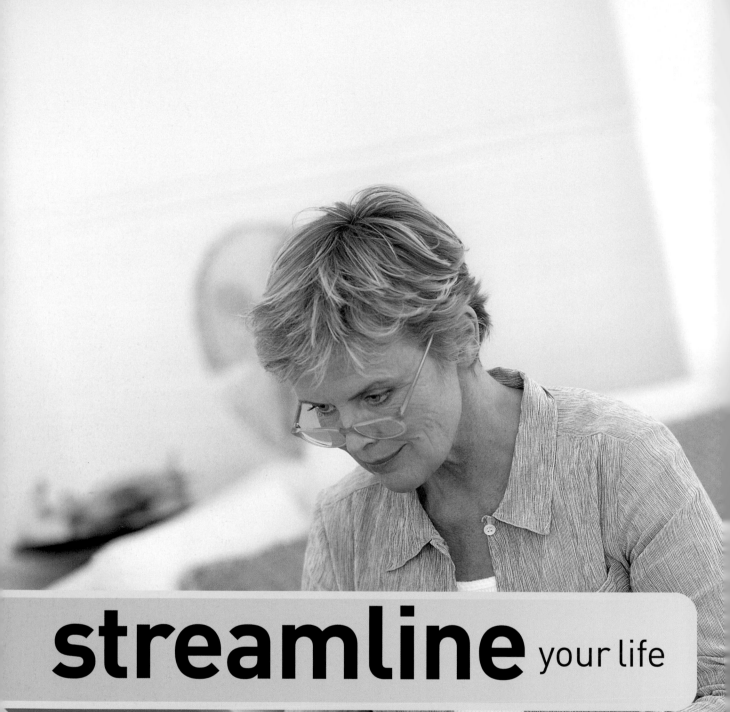
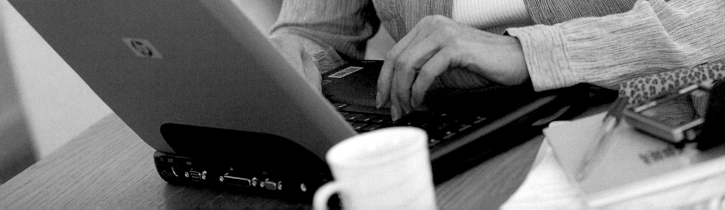

streamline your life

If you never have time to catch your breath, can't decide what to do first out of your long list of chores and rarely get a chance to even think – you need to streamline your life. It's easier than you might imagine.

While the later years of middle age can be relaxed and with plenty of 'me' time to spare, those in their 40s and early-to-mid 50s are more likely never to feel their feet touch the floor as they race through life, always seemingly one pace behind where they really need to be.

These years can be more time-poor than any other period. It is also true that the older we get the more quickly days, months and years seem to go by. This is because when you are, say, five years old, a year represents one-fifth of your whole life to date, and so seems a very long time. When you are 50, a year is only one-fiftieth of your whole life to date and so seems correspondingly shorter.

If you manage to find time to read Streamline Your Life it should help you save a great deal of time. If you often feel that your life is surrounded by chaos and muddle, you need it more than most.

We look at how to make each minute count by organizing your days, starting with the most important part of all – planning. This will improve your efficiency. We help you to redefine your priorities – weeding out the unnecessaries from your life and learning how to deal diplomatically with the time-wasting elements/people. We see how you can gain extra time by using a few sensible, but often overlooked, strategies. Finally, we look at how to be body-fit and brain-fit for 'extra time'.

Live by the Rules for Successful Time Management and … look … you can suddenly relax!

getting organized
Yes, it does sound boring, but if you want more time for your own needs you just have to get yourself organized. Think of it as freeing yourself up to be able to lead a better, more selfish (in the right sense) and more exciting life.

the importance of planning

First you need to plan ahead — for some reason, women are often better at this than men, but once men get the drift they can make excellent planners. Planning life just as you might make plans in your business is vital, for without it you just wake up in the morning and muddle your way through the day; or you start the week and muddle your way through that too. So if you are a person who feels that time spent thinking is time wasted, then DO think again. Sort your life out logically and you will no longer have to rush around.

Let's find an example. You need food for lunch, so you go to the shop and buy ingredients to make soup. Later on, you need food for supper, but you didn't get enough in the morning, so you have to go out again. Next day it is lunchtime and you have nothing to eat, but if you had cooked twice the amount of soup you would not have had to bother about lunch today. Extreme? No — when I'm away from home that is how my husband (dis)organizes his life all the time. But he has plenty of time to fill… Planning ahead could save him/you time both travelling, shopping and cooking.

how to plan Make schedules for work and for home life. For both, have a short-term and long-term list of things you have to do. Write the long-term list up once every few weeks in order of importance and tick items off when done. Write the short-term list every couple of days and similarly try to put the hardest/most important tasks first. Psychologically, this helps you to get them done.

Also, think about the order from a practical point of view. Do the chores meld into each other well and save you having to keep chopping and changing modes between them? Never make a journey (even a trip up the stairs at home) without seeing if it can't be used for more than one thing. Example: You go upstairs to find a different pair of shoes to wear. Take up the clean laundry as you go.

Never shop for the short term — buy as much as is practical every trip. Also have a 'fun' schedule. Decide on times during the day when you will have a relaxing break, or do some small selfish thing for yourself. If you don't schedule these in it is unlikely that you will do them.

prioritize

The next thing busy people are sometimes poor at is prioritizing. Here's another example. You've been working very long hours for weeks and weeks, seven days a week, to get a project done. You are exhausted and have had no social life at all. The phone rings. It is a teacher from your child's old school, asking if you will go and give a half-day talk to some pupils about a topic that you specialize in. What do you say? Well, you say 'yes', of course. Extreme? No — I did it myself not long ago. Why? Because it IS hard to say no. But sometimes you have to.

how to prioritize Spend a while with computer or paper and pen, prioritizing.

First your obligations. Make a list of things which are non-negotiable. These might be a certain number of hours at work, commuting, sleeping, showering, etc. Then a list of the things you have to do, but which you could spend less time on and get away with it. These might be, at home, cooking or housework, or, at work, checking e-mails or reading reports. In fact, if you work, make a separate list of how you might save time in the workplace. Unless you are tied to set hours, this will cut down the time you spend there. If you do have set hours, at least you will be less stressed out at work with fewer chores to do.

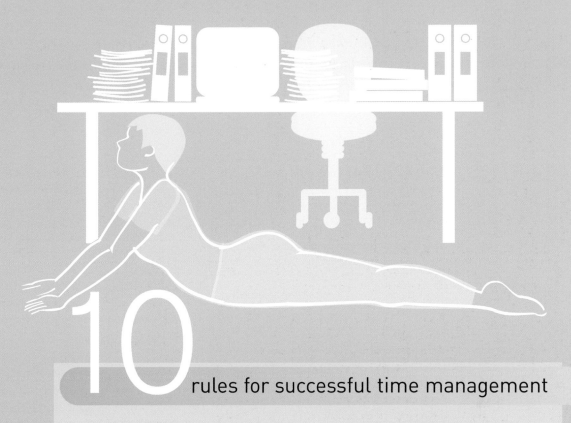

10 rules for successful time management

- Recognize the areas in which you are not being time-efficient.

- Prioritize using your own values, not someone else's.

- Never allow your time to be totally engulfed with work and obligations. Always factor in time for family, friends, leisure, health etc.

- Do harder or less welcome tasks early in the day – not only is your brain usually better able to cope at this time, but it also helps you to feel better about yourself, and therefore more efficient, for the remainder of the day.

- At the end of the day, know what you intend to do tomorrow. At the end of the week, know what you intend to do next week. This helps you to relax and unwind overnight/over the weekend. Even if things don't exactly go according to plan, at least you have a base from which to work.

- Don't aim for perfection. Aim to do as good a job on each task as you can reasonably expect in the time.

- When doing a task, focus 100% on it. It will get done quicker and better.

- Don't let pleasures become pressures too. When you feel that trip to the squash court or the drama club is too much like work, give it a rest.

- Always factor in 'chill' time every day. Sometimes you need to just do nothing.

- Use help when it is offered – and if it isn't offered, ask for it.

Cheer up – you DO have more time! Life is getting longer. In the UK, life expectancy is now 75 for men and 80 for women, and has doubled in the past 130 years. Positive thinking can also add years to your life – on average someone with a cheerful and positive outlook lives 7.5 years longer than a gloomy person.

Now a list of things you could get someone else to do. Delegate or pay someone else to do things, especially those that you are not so good at, or don't enjoy.

Then a list of things you do out of habit, but which may be a waste of your time. These might include watching TV every night (even the programmes you don't enjoy); reading trash magazines that other people bring home; surfing the Internet aimlessly; or lying too long in bed at the weekend. Decide what you could cut back on without loss of pleasure in life.

Lastly, make a list of things you do that you really don't want to do and which aren't necessary. This might include the talk at the school, chairing a local committee, keeping in touch with a friend you haven't really got on well with for years, and so on.

Now go through your lists and work out how much time you might save just on having the right priorities in life. You can now use some of the time you save on what you really want to do.

ways to make more time

Here we look at all the other factors apart from prioritizing and planning which may affect your ability to make the most of your time. You need energy. When you are feeling refreshed and full of energy you can skate through twice as much work/housework/reading etc. as when you are lethargic physically or mentally (it's hard to separate the two).

If you are physically fit – with both strength and stamina – you can, obviously, do physical work more quickly. Jobs like housework, gardening and shopping will all be easier to do. If your body is fit, your circulation will be in optimum shape, which, in turn, will mean that your brain works well (see opposite). Read Exercise for Energy (pages 86–9).

Watch your stress levels – although in the short-term stress can be a good thing and you may seem to have much more energy than usual because of the extra adrenaline it releases, if you are under constant stress in the long term your energy will suffer. For more on stress, see pages 202–3.

you need to think laterally You're energetic and organized – but you still don't seem to have enough time in the day. Try some of these ideas:

Pay! Recognize that you are not always the best person to do a task and don't feel guilty for employing help if you are time-poor. Never feel guilty for employing cleaners, window cleaners, child carers and so on. Even use a lifestyle manager if necessary (someone who will buy kid's clothes, presents, keep the household organized – in fact, do everything the old-fashioned 'wife and mother' – or, these days, 'househusband and father' – might have done.)

If you do have to provide meals either for yourself or a houseful, always buy ready-prepared vegetables, salads, cuts of meat, etc. Buy chilled-counter and deli goods rather than the more mass-market ready meals and ingredients. Buy luxury (oysters, caviar) or honest top-quality healthy foods (stone-baked breads, perfect olive oil) if you are time-poor. Complicated recipes may only be for people who don't buy the best!

Get multi-tasking You can talk, listen, write and think at the same time when you get used to it, especially if you are brain-fit (see opposite) and well rested (see Insomnia and sleep, pages 188–9).

Use white lies. It is easy to get a boring person, who is repeating themselves for the fifth time, off the telephone if you say you have to go because someone is at the door/has arrived for a meeting/you have to rush off etc. etc. In emergencies, disconnect your voice-mail and e-mail, which will save lots of time replying to messages left.

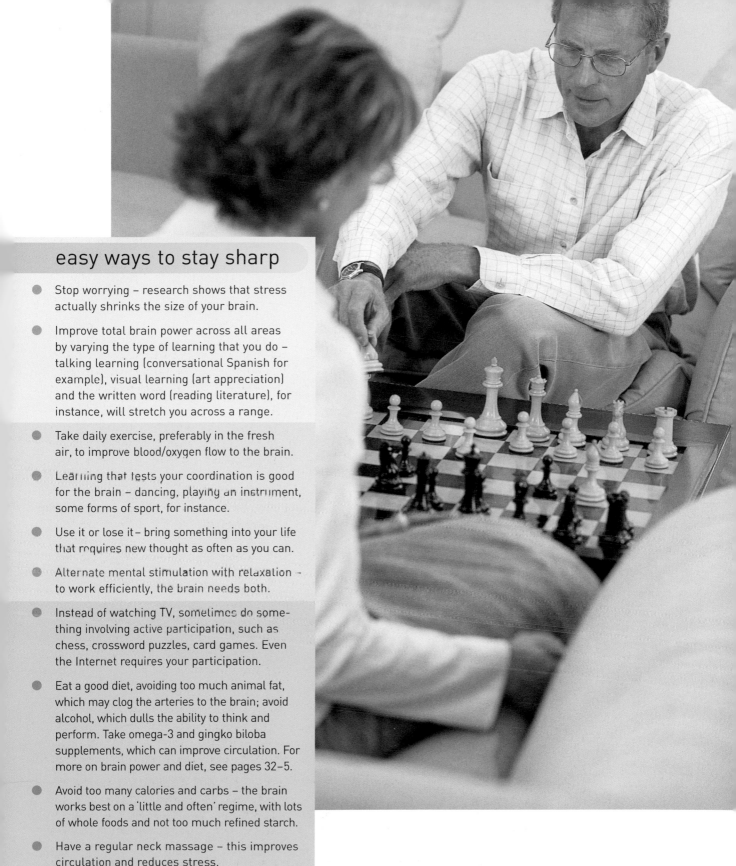

easy ways to stay sharp

- Stop worrying – research shows that stress actually shrinks the size of your brain.

- Improve total brain power across all areas by varying the type of learning that you do – talking learning (conversational Spanish for example), visual learning (art appreciation) and the written word (reading literature), for instance, will stretch you across a range.

- Take daily exercise, preferably in the fresh air, to improve blood/oxygen flow to the brain.

- Learning that tests your coordination is good for the brain – dancing, playing an instrument, some forms of sport, for instance.

- Use it or lose it – bring something into your life that requires new thought as often as you can.

- Alternate mental stimulation with relaxation – to work efficiently, the brain needs both.

- Instead of watching TV, sometimes do something involving active participation, such as chess, crossword puzzles, card games. Even the Internet requires your participation.

- Eat a good diet, avoiding too much animal fat, which may clog the arteries to the brain; avoid alcohol, which dulls the ability to think and perform. Take omega-3 and gingko biloba supplements, which can improve circulation. For more on brain power and diet, see pages 32–5.

- Avoid too many calories and carbs – the brain works best on a 'little and often' regime, with lots of whole foods and not too much refined starch.

- Have a regular neck massage – this improves circulation and reduces stress.

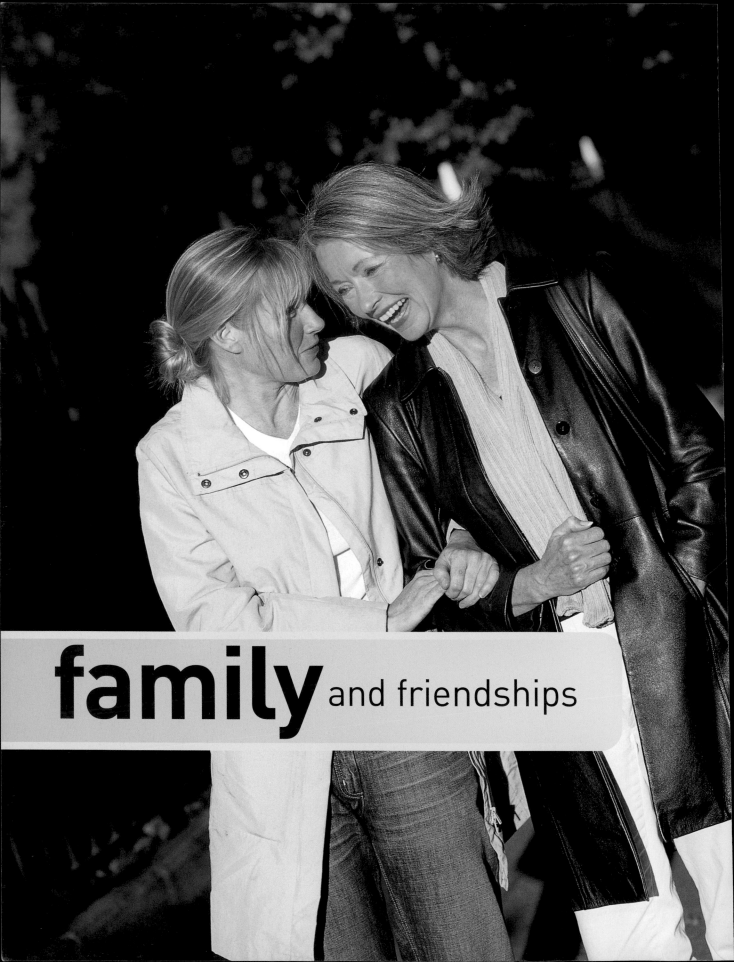

family and friendships

We are all guilty of neglecting our family and friends at least some of the time – and yet what they give us can be more enduring and fulfilling than any career; more comforting than any counsellor. Our relationships affect our happiness more than our bank balance does – and that's official, as discovered by the UK Economic and Social Research Council. Do you need to do some repair work?

The most important relationship most of us are likely to have is a marriage or other similar long-term commitment to another person. Indeed, plenty of research shows that people who are married tend to be happier and healthier than people who live alone. Surprising, then, that marriage is on the decrease, divorce is now commonplace and a large percentage of people over the age of 50 live on their own.

In this time-deficient twenty-first century world of rush, hustle, stress and travel, the state of friendship is also suffering. Long-term friendships are rarer than they were fifty years ago, with only a small minority of us still in touch with people we knew before the age of 20. We have acquaintances rather than deep friendships and people sometimes seem as disposable as a tissue.

And when we do know people well and/or in the long term, we tend to abuse those friendships, letting them slide, letting them fade and finally disappear. And perhaps we treat our life partners worst of all – having affairs, telling lies, taking them for granted… We have all done at least one of those three things.

Yet it is established that human beings are tribal creatures, we survive best with close and regular contact with others… relationships, friendships, physical contact, emotional closeness. Whether it is with partners, children, siblings, parents or friends – we cope better if people who know us are a permanent part of our lives.

In this final chapter we look at the complicated state of modern family relationships and friendships and see what sense we can make of it all.

partnerships

Marriage – or long-term living together – is something that, for those of us who have it, we either tend to take for granted, accepting grudgingly that it is OK, or kind of quietly wriggle and niggle and wonder what the hell we are doing with THIS person all this time. We wonder what are we missing.

No wonder so many marriages go awry in the middle years. The so-called mid-life crisis sees men and women disappearing off with younger partners, vanishing to go backpacking round the world, or simply to live alone and take up yoga and self-improvement courses. Most splits in partnerships aren't the result of one half of the partnership being wicked or cruel or robbing a bank, or even because of never-ending full-decibel rows or mental cruelty. Mostly the marriage just runs out of steam, with neither party bothering to invest enough effort to keep it going. Until finally the 'grass may be greener' philosophy provides the push.

the 4 stages of marriage

Psychologists describe four stages to the typical marriage. First, the romantic, lustful stage which lasts from 1 to 3 years. Next, the power struggle stage, when you both find your place in the marital pecking order and have bouts of thinking, 'What did I ever see in this person?' This lasts for the next 5 to 10 years. Towards the end of this stage you either split up, reach a compromise or, occasionally, find that you both want the same things out of life and each other and are blissfully 'happily married'.

The third stage, which comes along gradually, is the 'completely taking each other for granted' stage, when your sex life often virtually comes to a halt and the partner is part of the furniture, and you accept – but sometimes despise – that person, warts and all. Or occasionally you simply put up with him or her until the kids have left home and you can be off. This stage is obviously vulnerable to either partner having affairs to reaffirm their attractiveness and as an outlet for sex. Stage three can last up twenty years or more, but in a positive marriage may be much shorter or non-existent.

Lastly, should you by any chance get through all that, and learn the lesson that perhaps your partner is quite nice after all – and that there isn't all that much time left to argue – you have the 'reward' stage: two people living their peaceful – or sometimes even exciting – years together as friends, partners and lovers in the true sense, sometimes still with a hint of sex there, but if not it doesn't matter. All is well in the world. Sadly only half of all couples reach that stage – or they continue living in Stage Three, until one dies or bails out.

Assuming you have got through stages one and two and are still married but feel that things could be better – what can you do to keep the partnership going? First, ask yourself whether you have a basic foundation to the marriage so that it is worth working on. When the children have left home is often a good time to do this. If there are grounds for serious complaints on either side – you feel trapped, perhaps, in a marriage that is enslaving, restricting or oppressive, for instance – these need to be worked out before you can begin improvements.

Sometimes this will need the help of a relationship counsellor, because, if you haven't talked together for years, it is really hard to begin what can often be awkward conversations, bringing up things that have remained unsaid for years, on your own. Next, should there be any causes for forgiveness, these need to be addressed. Affairs and major fall-outs should be put behind you and forgiven if not completely forgotten.

If your sex life is not what you both want, then see the chapter on Libido or, again, seek counselling. Should you both have been taking each other for granted, in one way that isn't such a bad thing, but you need to begin valuing your partner again. Writing a list of their good points is a good start.

Their faults? If there are any you still find hard to accept after all this time, perhaps they could be discussed – although asking someone to stop leaving the top off the toothpaste after thirty years may not get you far. Some habits and personality traits can't be changed – however, research shows people do evolve, and many things can be improved if you encourage without nagging. You have to accept that your partner should do the same to you … and that all people come with traits you may perceive as faults. Not expecting too much is a hard lesson, but it can be the making of your marriage, even after many years.

Long-term prospects of roses round the door at 80? Do you like that person? Do you want to share most of your time with them? Do you have enough in common? Do you like your life with that person? If mostly yes, then stay with it. 60% of people who get divorced later say they regret it. A marriage that has lasted 20, 25, 30 years is worth fighting for.

If not, there is no disgrace in splitting up/divorcing/separating, or of living next door to each other and being friends. People find their own ways; there are no clear-cut rules.

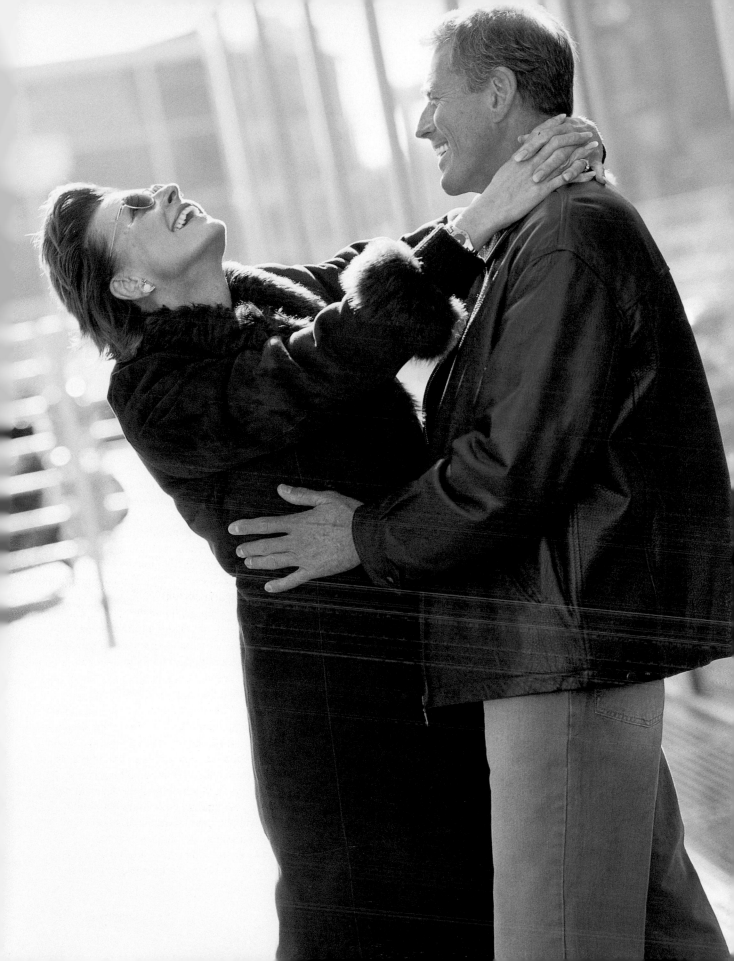

family
Disagreements between couples over how to treat the children can do as much serious harm to a marriage during mid life as they can when the children are very small. And conflict between parents and children, as well as you and your own parents, can also disrupt the household – or at least your peace of mind.

Now couples are having their children later – in their mid-to-late thirties is quite commonplace – this means that the 50s, which were once the decade for peace, prosperity and selfish pleasures, are the most manic of all our lives. Teenagers on the loose! Moods! Drugs! Mess! Transport disagreements! Noise! Sex! Love angst! And then it's university problems, money worries, more drugs, alcohol, more love angst, malnutrition … Why did you have them? Why do you put up with it? Because you love them.

The trick with teens still at home is to have a strong belief that this will pass, for it will. They will, sooner rather than later in most cases, turn into lovely – or at least passable – human beings. The second trick is not to let them ruin your relationship with your partner. 'Divide and rule' is their motto – don't let it happen. Single parents have the advantage here. Couples need to talk to each other about their children before they talk to the children – that way, if one of you disagrees on a course of action you work it out before the child realizes they may be able to milk the situation.

The third motto is to get and/or keep a life of your own. The one thing teens and early 20s hate more than anything is to have to feel responsible, guilty or worried about you – they have enough trouble worrying about themselves. If you can be seen to be being happy and enjoying life, they will like that. But don't overdo it – they also want you to be there when it is important.

Forget sending them food parcels twice a week or worrying about their laundry – that is their problem. But you need to give the impression you are somewhere in the background, caring about them and hoping they are happy. Laid-back love, something like that. They also need to know they can come back to the family home at any time, once they have left – but not to sponge off you.

Avoid, at all costs, meddling, alienating them and their friends/lovers, competing for their affections and time, taking sides when there is more than one sibling, and being overprotective.

parents and dependants
Sometimes life doesn't seem fair. When breathing that big sigh of relief because the kids have finally left home or are at least showing signs of independence, you are faced with an elderly parent or in-law who can't cope on their own. Do you invite them into your house/convert the shed? Do you recognize caring for them as your duty or do you put them in the nearest care home and stick to the Sunday visit?

My view is that you should put your partner and children first and your parent second. That means discussing the situation with your own family and seeing what their views are and then, if possible, finding a solution which is acceptable to all. Never decide that a parent or relative can come to live with you unless you are as near 100% sure as you can be that you will be able to stay the course. If taking them in will lead to divorce, it is not the right decision.

If it really isn't possible for the dependant to come and live with you – and, after all, many families don't have room – then managed accommodation or a care home is the obvious answer. Get an appointment with your local social services to talk through all the problems and questions you have surrounding this decision, and you should make sure that the dependant understands all the way along what is happening, as far as that is possible.

One last alternative is to share the care among you and your siblings (or the in-law siblings), which would mean the dependant moving home every few months or so.

Once a decision is made after careful thought and planning – don't feel guilty.

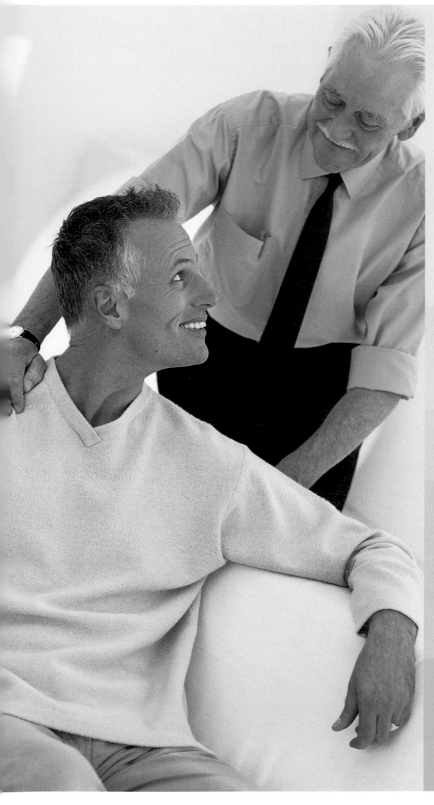

can they live with you?

- If your dependants are ill or infirm you may not be able to provide the care necessary. In that case you need to see what care and nursing help you can expect in the home, and what respite care will be on offer.

- Although you may feel sorry – and perhaps responsible – for that person, if you never got along with them all through your lives, it is unlikely that you will get on with them now.

- People who are dependent do tend to get crustier, not sweeter. This is worth bearing in mind.

- If you live with a relative, don't let them 'rule the roost' by emotional blackmail or any other means. Any children left at home, as well as you and your partner, need to have a quality of life too.

- Consider your own personality, and the commitments you already have in place. Do you have the time and energy to do this extra work?

- Don't feel angry if your partner feels he or she can't live with the relative in question – it isn't an obligation of modern marriage and you shouldn't feel aggrieved if this is the case.

- Are there any other people who have, morally, as big a responsibility towards the care of this person as you do – e.g. other brothers, sisters etc.? If so, why are you taking it as your problem alone?

- Will there be advantages that are important to you or others in the household apart from the dependant? For example, if you all get on well it might be an even happier household; by taking in that person you may feel more comfortable with yourself, and so on.

firming up your friendships
From the cradle to the grave, you need friends – and mid life is the perfect time to reassess your friendships ... affirming current ones, renewing old acquaintances and even making new pals to see you through the next fifty years or so.

When you were little, you were never happier than when you had a 'best friend' to play with. When you were a teenager, you wanted to be one of 'the gang'. In your 20s you probably had a few close friends and were adept at making new ones, while beginning to realize that friendships can easily fade away if you don't invest time in them. By the middle years, some of us have a wide circle of good friends, many kept since those early years. But others of us have managed to lose most of them along the years by putting work or family first.

If you're feeling now that you wish you'd invested more effort or time on developing, nurturing and keeping friends, don't worry – it isn't too late to do something about it. No need for desperate measures – like a neighbour of mine who every Christmas gets out all her old cards and puts them up, or the work colleague who leaves messages for herself on her voice-mail at home so she won't feel depressed when she gets in.

reaffirming current friendships
Old, long-standing friends are a bit like marriage partners – we tend to take them for granted. This is fine up to a point – but you can't sustain a real friendship if you invest no effort for years. Friendships need feeding.

First write a list of your current friends. Not acquaintances from work or neighbours you say 'Hi' to – proper friends. A recent UK survey found the average Briton claims 14 friends, but I feel this is a bit of an exaggeration – like the surveys on sex where we all claim to do it twice a night, every night at the age of 60. We don't want to admit the truth sometimes!

If you can write down several, good. It doesn't have to be 14. Think about each one, when you last contacted them, how much time you spend 'interacting'. If you feel you have been remiss in keeping that friendship alive, do something about it. But only do this if you really do want to keep in touch with that person.

For friendship to work at any age, the friend needs to bring something that you need to the relationship. That's why having different types of friends usually works best. One for golf, one for drinking, one for going to the theatre, one for gossiping, one for moaning, and, if you're married, a few communal marriage couple friends… you know the sort of thing. If all your friends come into the same group (all golfing cronies, for instance) consider expanding your repertoire.

If at this stage you are wondering whether you are potentially popular enough to win over all these new friends, don't worry. Of course you are. Popularity is nothing more than giving people what they need. All the people you tend to like best as friends are those who make YOU feel good, either about yourself, or about life. That, or they affirm who you are and that others feel the same way as you. So, you do that for other people, and you will be perennially popular.

Having money can work against you more than having no money. If you are wealthy, don't slosh the cash around and don't boast. Nice people are sometimes intimidated by signs of affluence. And you don't want the kind of 'friends' who think you will dip your hand in your pocket all the time.

renewing old friendships
Don't feel embarrassed about contacting someone you haven't seen or spoken to for years. It happens to everyone. Every single person goes through life and loses friends – we move, we get busy, we change. But something strange happens in mid life – we begin to think about the people we used to know at school, at college, at our first workplace, in our old home town. Think about the people you used to like. Chances are you will still like them, even if you have both changed outwardly.

Friendships that lapsed more recently can also sometimes be revived – it is quite likely that the person you contact will be delighted to be in touch again. If not – well, you've lost nothing; at least you tried. Give it a go – make contact by e-mail, card or phone. You may still have a great deal to offer each other.

making new friends
Why do people think that as they get older they won't be able to make new friends? Or that they don't want new friends? Yes, it's wonderful to have a cache of people we've known for years, who know us inside out, but you should carry on bringing people into your life even at 90. They give you a new view on the world, and make you take a new look at yourself, too.

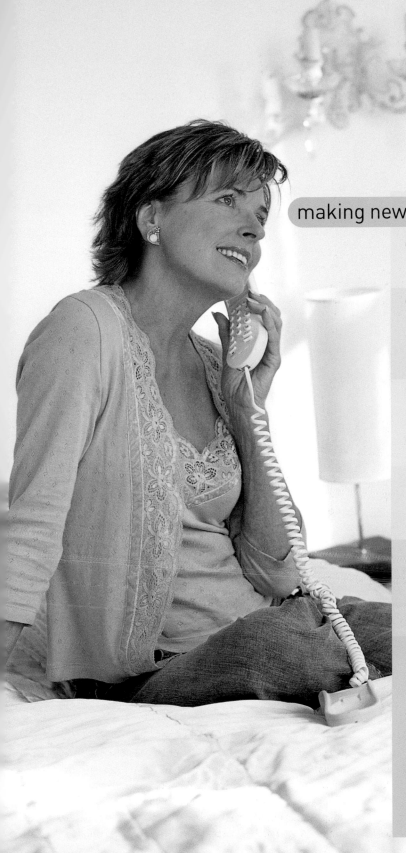

making new friends and keeping old ones

- Someone has to make the first move – why not you? You are unlikely to make friends sitting in front of the TV.

- In the early stages of a friendship, people are often attracted to someone who makes them feel that life can be wonderful – so talk yourself and your life up a little and try to be upbeat most of the time. Make 'em laugh.

- The most effective way to start a friendship with someone you already know a little is an offer of help, be it knowledge ('I have a book at home that will help'), practical ('let me drive you to the station') or emotional support.

- Another good way is to offer the chance of a shared experience –'I have a spare ticket to the concert – would you like to come?' or 'Are you going to the open day – shall we go together?'

- Don't bombard people with phone calls, visits, etc. Take your time – people like to slide naturally into new friendships.

- Don't be upset if things don't work out. You can't like everyone and they can't all like you.

- To be a friend, a person doesn't have to share all your likes and dislikes. Be tolerant.

- If you have a misunderstanding or disagreement, get it sorted quickly.

- Give people the benefit of the doubt and don't expect perfection. No one is perfect.

- Remember your friends have other friends too. Don't take it personally if a friend invites someone else out, or if they can't take up an invitation from you because they are busy.

addresses and contacts

NOTE: When writing to organizations to request information, please enclose a stamped self-addressed, envelope.

fuel for your new life

British Dietetic Association
5th Floor,
Charles House,
148–149 Queensway,
Birmingham B3 3HT
Tel 0121 200 8080
www.bda.uk.com

British Nutrition Foundation
52–54 High Holborn,
London WC1V 6RQ
Tel 020 7210 4850
www.nutrition.org.uk

The Food Commission
94 White Lion Street,
London N1 9PF
Tel 020 7837 2250
www.foodcomm.org.uk

Food Standards Agency
Aviation House,
125 Kingsway,
London WC2B 6NH
Tel 020 7276 8000
www.foodstandards.gov.uk

Weight Watchers UK Ltd
Ludlow Road,
Maidenhead, Berks SL6 2SL
Tel 0845 345 1500
www.weightwatchers.co.uk

Women's Nutritional Advisory Service
PO Box 268,
Lewes, East Sussex BN7 1QN
Tel 012173 487366
www.wnas.org.uk

body for your new life

Exercise classes, gyms and health clubs
www.Gymuser.co.uk

National Register of Personal Trainers
0870 200 6010
www.nrpt.co.uk

Society of Teachers of the Alexander Technique
20 London House,
266 Fulham Road
London SW10 9EL
Tel 020 7284 3338
www.stat.org.uk

pilates
Body Control Pilates information line:
0870 16900000
www.bodycontrol.co.uk
www.pilatesfoundation.com

British Wheel of Yoga
1 Hamilton Place,
Boston Rd, Sleaford
Lincs NG34 7ES
Tel: 01529 306851
www.bwy.org.uk

National Back Pain Association
Tel 020 8977 5474
www.backpain.org/

Ramblers Association
Tel: 020 7339 8500
www.ramblers.co.uk

looks for your new life

British Association of Aesthetic Plastic Surgeons
Royal College of Surgeons
33–43 Lincoln's Inn Fields,
London WC2A 3PN
Tel 020 7405 2234

American Society of Plastic Surgeons
Tel 1-888-475-2784
www.plasticsurgery.org/

Institute of Trichologists
Hairdressing and Beauty Industry Authority
Tel 01302 380000
www.habia.org.uk

Discounted designer clothes
www.yellowsearch.co.uk
www.uksites.net/clothes.htm

well-being for your new life

Cancer Bacup
Helpline 0808 800 1234
www.cancerbacup.org.uk

Diabetes UK
10 Queen Anne Street,
London W1G 9LH
Tel: 020 7323 1531
www.diabetes.org.uk

The British Menopause Society
www.the-bms.org/

The Menopause Amarant Trust
Tel 020 7401 3855
www.amarantmenopause.org.uk/

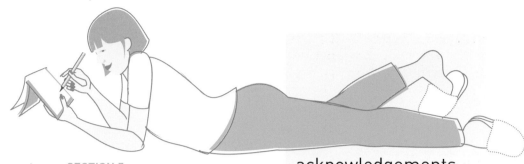

British Association for Counselling and Psychotherapy
1 Regent Place,
Rugby,
Warks CV21 2PJ
Tel: 0870 4435252
www.bacp.co.uk

British Association for Behavioural and Cognitive Psychotherapy
PO Box 9,
Accrington,
Lancs BB5 2GD
Tel 01254 875277

MIND (National Association for Mental Health)
Tel 0845 766 0163
www.mind.org.uk

Relate
Telephone 0845 130 4010
www.relate.co.uk

National Osteoporosis Society
Camerton,
Bath BA2 OPJ
Tel 01761 471771
www.nos.org.uk

The British Massage Therapy Council
17 Rymers Lane,
Oxford OX4 3JU
Tel 01865 774123
www.bmtc.co.uk

British Heart Foundation
14 Fitzhardinge Street,
London W1H 4DH
Tel: 020 7935 0185
www.bhf.org.uk

IBS Network
Northern General Hospital,
Sheffield S5 7AU
Tel 0114 261153

SECTION 5
time for your new life

National Association of Bereavement Services
20 Norton Folgate,
London E1 6DB
Tel 020 7247 1080

Dating
www.speeddater.co.uk

Friends Reunited
www.friendsreunited.co.uk

Maturity Works
Tel 020 8667 0175
www.maturityworks.co.uk

Work-Life Balance Trust
www.w-lb.org.uk

Association of Retired and Persons Over 50
Tel 020 8683 8998
www.arp050.org.uk

Third Age Employment Network
Tel 020 8843 1590
www.taen.org.uk

The Third Age
Tel 020 8466 6139
www.u3a.org.uk

Executives Recycled
Tel 08707 653821
www.executives-recycled.co.uk

Saga
Saga Building,
Middelburg Street,
Folkestone,
Kent CT20 1AZ
Tel 0800 414 525
01303 771 111
www.saga.co.uk

acknowledgements

All photographs © **Liz McAulay**

except the front cover © John Powell/Retna UK; pages 9, 15, 18 and 35 © Robert Harding Picture Library; and page 20 © Digital Vision.

The publisher would like to thank the following for their generosity in supplying items of clothing for photography: Next (daywear), Marks & Spencer (sportswear and underwear) and Frank Usher (evening wear).

Thanks also to the models: from CLOSE Management Ltd – Sarah Bee and her son, Francine Bloom, Suzi Conway and Janie Simmonds – and at MOT Models – Mike Morrell, Greg Sherriff, Tiffany Suchard and Joanna Woodley. And to the make-up artists: from Joy Goodman – James McMahon and Dottie Monaghan.

The author would like to express her thanks to the following people for their invaluable input and help in making this book possible: Lewis Esson, Mary Evans, Jane Turnbull, Jane O'Shea and all the rest of the team at Quadrille.

index